ABC OF
INTERVENTIONAL CARDIOLOGY

For Lisa, Alexander, and Frances

ABC OF
INTERVENTIONAL CARDIOLOGY

Edited by

EVER D GRECH
Consultant Cardiologist, South Yorkshire Cardiothoracic Centre,
Northern General Hospital, Sheffield, UK

First published in 2004
by BMJ Publishing Group Ltd, BMA House, Tavistock Square,
London WC1H 9JR

www.bmjbooks.com

British Library Cataloguing in Publication Data
A catalogue record for this book is available from the British Library

ISBN 0 7279 1546 0

Cover shows coloured arteriogram of arteries of the heart.
With permission from Science Photo Library.

Typeset by BMJ Electronic Production and Newgen Imaging Systems
Printed and bound in Spain by GraphyCems, Navarra

Contents

Contributors

David Crossman
Professor of Clinical Cardiology, Cardiovascular Research Group, Clinical Sciences Centre, Northern General Hospital, Sheffield

David Cumberland
Consultant Cardiovascular Interventionist, Ampang Puteri Specialist Hospital, Kuala Lumpur, Malaysia

John Ducas
Consultant Cardiologist, Health Sciences Centre and St Boniface Hospital, Winnipeg, Manitoba and Associate Professor, University of Manitoba, Winnipeg, Canada

Ever D Grech
Consultant Cardiologist, South Yorkshire Cardiothoracic Centre, Northern General Hospital, Sheffield, UK

Julian Gunn
Senior Lecturer and Honorary Consultant Cardiologist, Cardiovascular Research Group, Clinical Sciences Centre, Northern General Hospital, Sheffield

Timothy Houghton
Registrar in Cardiology, Hull and East Yorkshire Trust, Castle Hill Hospital, Hull

Gerry C Kaye
Consultant Cardiologist, Hull and East Yorkshire Trust, Castle Hill Hospital, Hull

Laurence O'Toole
Consultant Cardiologist and Physician, Royal Hallamshire Hospital, Sheffield

Roger Philipp
Fellow in Interventional Cardiology, Health Sciences Centre and St Boniface Hospital, Winnipeg, Manitoba, Canada

David R Ramsdale
Consultant Cardiologist, Cardiothoracic Centre, Liverpool

Kevin P Walsh
Consultant Paediatric Cardiologist, Our Lady's Hospital for Sick Children, Crumlin, Dublin, Republic of Ireland

Preface

It is only 26 years since the first percutaneous transluminal coronary angioplasty (PTCA) was carried out by the pioneering Swiss radiologist, Andreas Greuntzig, heralding the dawn of interventional cardiology. In this short time, interventional cardiology has overcome many limitations and undergone major evolutionary changes—most notably the development of the coronary stent. Worldwide, many thousands of patients now safely undergo percutaneous coronary intervention every day, and the numbers continue to grow. In many countries, the numbers are similar to, or exceed, bypass surgical procedures.

Although, at first, PTCA was indicated only as treatment for chronic stable angina caused by a discrete lesion in a single vessel, this has now progressed to encompass multi-lesion and multi-vessel disease. Moreover, percutaneous intervention is now becoming widely used in the management of unstable angina and acute myocardial infarction with definite benefits in terms of morbidity and mortality. The effectiveness and safety of these procedures has undoubtedly been enhanced by the adjunctive use of new anti-platelet and antithrombotic agents.

As the indications increase and more patients are treated, so inevitably do the demands on healthcare budgets. Undoubtedly, percutaneous intervention is expensive. However, this burden must be weighed against bypass surgery, which is even more costly, and multi-drug treatment—which would be required over many years.

Although percutaneous coronary intervention has held centre stage in cardiology, major in-roads have also been made in non-coronary areas. Transcatheter valvuloplasty, ethanol septal ablation and closure devices have become effective and safe alternatives to surgery, as have paediatric interventional procedures. A greater understanding of cardiac electrophysiology has led to important advances in the treatment of arrhythmias, and implantable cardioverter defibrillators are benefiting ever larger numbers of patients.

Where are we heading? This is perhaps the biggest question in the minds of many interventional cardiologists. New technology generated by industry and new techniques coupled with high levels of expertise are fuelling advances in almost all areas of interventional cardiology. As drug-eluting stents address the Achilles' heel of angioplasty and stenting—restenosis—the huge increase in percutaneous coronary procedures seen over recent years is likely to increase even further, and will probably be double the rate of bypass surgery within a decade.

In writing and editing this book, I have endeavoured to present broad (and sometimes complex) aspects of interventional cardiology in a clear, concise and balanced manner. To this end, an easy-to-read style of text, avoiding jargon and exhaustive detail, has been used supplemented with many images and graphics.

EVER D GRECH
Sheffield, July 2003

Acknowledgements

I have many people to thank for helping me develop and produce this book. I am very grateful to my coauthors who have all willingly contributed their time and expertise. I would also like to recognise the positive efforts and invaluable assistance of the *British Medical Journal* editors and illustrators. These include Trish Groves, Mary Banks, Eleanor Lines, Greg Cotton, and Naomi Wilkinson.

Finally, my enduring gratitude goes to my family for their unfailing encouragement, patience, and love.

1 Pathophysiology and investigation of coronary artery disease

Ever D Grech

In affluent societies, coronary artery disease causes severe disability and more death than any other disease, including cancer. It manifests as angina, silent ischaemia, unstable angina, myocardial infarction, arrhythmias, heart failure, and sudden death.

Pathophysiology

Coronary artery disease is almost always due to atheromatous narrowing and subsequent occlusion of the vessel. Early atheroma (from the Greek athera (porridge) and oma (lump)) is present from young adulthood onwards. A mature plaque is composed of two constituents, each associated with a particular cell population. The lipid core is mainly released from necrotic "foam cells"—monocyte derived macrophages, which migrate into the intima and ingest lipids. The connective tissue matrix is derived from smooth muscle cells, which migrate from the media into the intima, where they proliferate and change their phenotype to form a fibrous capsule around the lipid core.

When a plaque produces a $>50\%$ diameter stenosis (or $>75\%$ reduction in cross sectional area), reduced blood flow through the coronary artery during exertion may lead to angina. Acute coronary events usually arise when thrombus formation follows disruption of a plaque. Intimal injury causes denudation of the thrombogenic matrix or lipid pool and triggers thrombus formation. In acute myocardial infarction, occlusion is more complete than in unstable angina, where arterial occlusion is usually subtotal. Downstream embolism of thrombus may also produce microinfarcts.

Investigations

Patients presenting with chest pain may be identified as having definite or possible angina from their history alone. In the former group, risk factor assessment should be undertaken, both to guide diagnosis and because modification of some associated risk factors can reduce cardiovascular events and mortality. A blood count, biochemical screen, and thyroid function tests may identify extra factors underlying the onset of angina. Initial drug treatment should include aspirin, a β blocker, and a nitrate. Antihypertensive and lipid lowering drugs may also be given, in conjunction with advice on lifestyle and risk factor modification.

All patients should be referred to a cardiologist to clarify the diagnosis, optimise drug treatment, and assess the need and suitability for revascularisation (which can improve both symptoms and prognosis). Patients should be advised to seek urgent medical help if their symptoms occur at rest or on minimal exertion and if they persist for more than 10 minutes after sublingual nitrate has been taken, as these may herald the onset of an acute coronary syndrome.

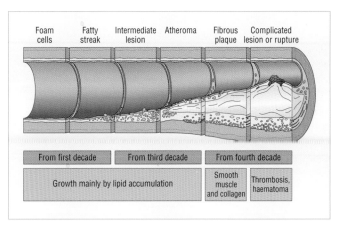

Progression of atheromatous plaque from initial lesion to complex and ruptured plaque

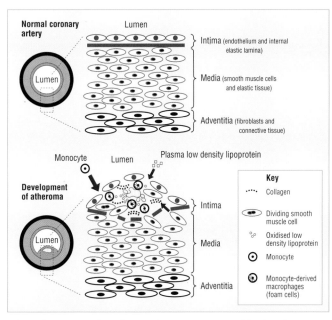

Schematic representation of normal coronary artery wall (top) and development of atheroma (bottom)

Priorities for cardiology referral

- Recent onset of symptoms
- Rapidly progressive symptoms
- Possible aortic stenosis
- Threatened employment
- Severe symptoms (minimal exertion or nocturnal angina)
- Angina refractory to medical treatment

Cardiovascular risk factors

Non-modifiable risk factors
- Positive family history
- Age
- Male sex

Modifiable risk factors
- Hypercholesterolaemia
- Left ventricular hypertrophy
- Overweight and obesity
- Hypertension
- Sedentary lifestyle
- Excessive alcohol intake
- Smoking
- Diabetes

Uncertain risk factors
- Hypertriglyceridaemia
- Microalbuminuria
- Hyperhomocysteinaemia
- Lp(a) lipoprotein
- Fibrinogen
- C reactive protein
- Uric acid
- Renin

1

Non-invasive investigations

Electrocardiography

An abnormal electrocardiogram increases the suspicion of significant coronary disease, but a normal result does not exclude it.

Chest x ray

Patients with angina and no prior history of cardiac disease usually have a normal chest x ray film.

Exercise electrocardiography

This is the most widely used test in evaluating patients with suspected angina. It is generally safe (risk ratio of major adverse events 1 in 2500, and of mortality 1 in 10 000) and provides diagnostic as well as prognostic information. The average sensitivity and specificity is 75%. The test is interpreted in terms of achieved workload, symptoms, and electrocardiographic response. A 1 mm depression in the horizontal ST segment is the usual cut-off point for significant ischaemia. Poor exercise capacity, an abnormal blood pressure response, and profound ischaemic electrocardiographic changes are associated with a poor prognosis.

Main end points for exercise electrocardiography

- Target heart rate achieved (>85% of maximum predicted heart rate)
- ST segment depression >1 mm (downsloping or planar depression of greater predictive value than upsloping depression)
- Slow ST recovery to normal (>5 minutes)
- Decrease in systolic blood pressure >20 mm Hg
- Increase in diastolic blood pressure >15 mm Hg
- Progressive ST segment elevation or depression
- ST segment depression >3 mm without pain
- Arrhythmias (atrial fibrillation, ventricular tachycardia)

Features indicative of a strongly positive exercise test

- Exercise limited by angina to <6 minutes of Bruce protocol
- Failure of systolic blood pressure to increase >10 mm Hg, or fall with evidence of ischaemia
- Widespread marked ST segment depression >3 mm
- Prolonged recovery time of ST changes (>6 minutes)
- Development of ventricular tachycardia
- ST elevation in absence of prior myocardial infarction

Stress echocardiography

Stress induced impairment of myocardial contraction is a sensitive marker of ischaemia and precedes electrocardiographic changes and angina. Cross sectional echocardiography can be used to evaluate regional and global left ventricular impairment during ischaemia, which can be induced by exercise or an intravenous infusion of drugs that increase myocardial contraction and heart rate (such as dobutamine) or dilate coronary arterioles (such as dipyridamole or adenosine). The test has a higher sensitivity and specificity than exercise electrocardiography and is useful in patients whose physical condition limits exercise.

Radionuclide myocardial perfusion imaging

Thallium-201 or technetium-99m (^{99m}Tc-sestamibi, ^{99m}Tc-tetrofosmin) is injected intravenously at peak stress, and its myocardial distribution relates to coronary flow. Images are acquired with a gamma camera. This test can distinguish between reversible and irreversible ischaemia (the latter signifying infarcted tissue). Although it is expensive and requires specialised equipment, it is useful in patients whose exercise test is non-diagnostic or whose exercise ability is limited.

Exercise stress testing

Indications

- Confirmation of suspected angina
- Evaluation of extent of myocardial ischaemia and prognosis
- Risk stratification after myocardial infarction
- Detection of exercise induced symptoms (such as arrhythmias or syncope)
- Evaluation of outcome of interventions (such as percutaneous coronary interventions or coronary artery bypass surgery)
- Assessment of cardiac transplant
- Rehabilitation and patient motivation

Contraindications

- Cardiac failure
- Any feverish illness
- Left ventricular outflow tract obstruction or hypertrophic cardiomyopathy
- Severe aortic or mitral stenosis
- Uncontrolled hypertension
- Pulmonary hypertension
- Recent myocardial infarction
- Severe tachyarrhythmias
- Dissecting aortic aneurysm
- Left main stem stenosis or equivalent
- Complete heart block (in adults)

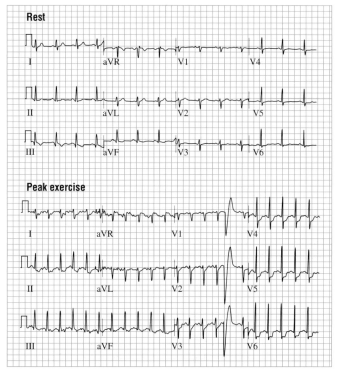

Example of a strongly positive exercise test. After only 2 minutes and 24 seconds of exercise (according to Bruce protocol), the patient developed chest pain and electrocardiography showed marked ischaemic changes (maximum 3 mm ST segment depression in lead V6)

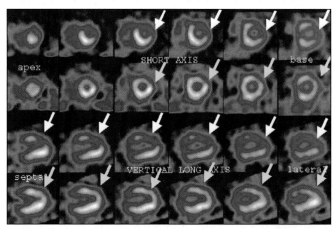

^{99m}Tc-tetrofosmin perfusion scan showing reversible anterolateral wall ischaemia, induced by intravenous dobutamine infusion (white arrows). Normal rest images are shown by yellow arrows

A multigated acquisition (MUGA) scan assesses left ventricular function and can reveal salvageable myocardium in patients with chronic coronary artery disease. It can be performed with either thallium scintigraphy at rest or metabolic imaging with fluorodeoxyglucose by means of either positron emission tomography (PET) or single photon emission computed tomography (SPECT).

Invasive investigations

Coronary angiography

The only absolute way to evaluate coronary artery disease is by angiography. It is usually performed as part of cardiac catheterisation, which includes left ventricular angiography and haemodynamic measurements, providing a more complete evaluation of an individual's cardiac status. Cardiac catheterisation is safely performed as a day case procedure.

Patients must be fully informed of the purpose of the procedure as well as its risks and limitations. Major complications, though rare in experienced hands, include death (risk ratio 1 in 1400), stroke (1 in 1000), coronary artery dissection (1 in 1000), and arterial access complications (1 in 500). Risks depend on the individual patient, and predictors include age, coronary anatomy (such as severe left main stem disease), impaired left ventricular function, valvar heart disease, the clinical setting, and non-cardiac disease. The commonest complications are transient or minor and include arterial access bleeding and haematoma, pseudoaneurysm, arrhythmias, reactions to the contrast medium, and vagal reactions (during sheath insertion or removal).

Before the procedure, patients usually fast and may be given a sedative. Although a local anaesthetic is used, arterial access (femoral, brachial, or radial) may be mildly uncomfortable. Patients do not usually feel the catheters once they are inside the arteries. Transient angina may occur during injection of contrast medium, usually because of a severely diseased artery. Patients should be warned that, during left ventricular angiography, the large volume of contrast medium may cause a transient hot flush and a strange awareness of urinary incontinence (and can be reassured that this does not actually happen). Modern contrast agents rarely cause nausea and vomiting.

Insertion of an arterial sheath with a haemostatic valve minimises blood loss and allows catheter exchange. Three types of catheter, which come in a variety of shapes and diameters, are commonly used. Two have a single hole at the end and are designed to facilitate controlled engagement of the distal tip within the coronary artery ostium. Contrast medium is injected through the lumen of the catheter, and moving x ray images are obtained and recorded. Other catheters may be used for graft angiography. The "pigtail" catheter has an end hole and several side holes and is passed across the aortic valve into the left ventricle. It allows injection of 30-40 ml of contrast medium

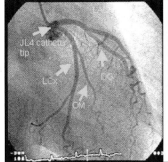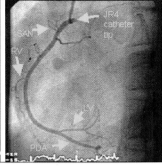

Angiograms of normal coronary arteries (LAD=left anterior descending artery, DG=diagonal artery, LCx=left circumflex artery, OM=obtuse marginal artery, SAN=sino-atrial node artery, RV=right ventricular branch artery, LV=left ventricular branch artery, PDA=posterior descending artery)

Main indications for coronary angiography

- Uncertain diagnosis of angina (coronary artery disease cannot be excluded by non-invasive testing)
- Assessment of feasibility and appropriateness of various forms of treatment (percutaneous intervention, bypass surgery, medical)
- Class I or II stable angina with positive stress test or class III or IV angina without positive stress test
- Unstable angina or non-Q wave myocardial infarction (medium and high risk patients)
- Angina not controlled by drug treatment
- Acute myocardial infarction—especially cardiogenic shock, ineligibility for thrombolytic treatment, failed thrombolytic reperfusion, re-infarction, or positive stress test
- Life threatening ventricular arrhythmia
- Angina after bypass surgery or percutaneous intervention
- Before valve surgery or corrective heart surgery to assess occult coronary artery disease

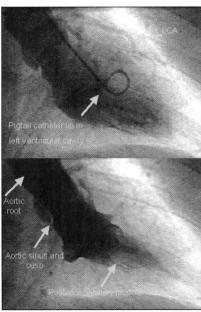

Left ventricular angiogram during diastole (top) and systole (bottom) after injection of contrast medium via a pigtail catheter, showing good contractility (LCA=left coronary artery)

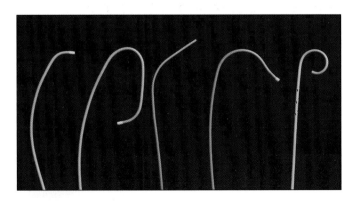

Commonly used diagnostic catheters (from left to right): right Judkins, left Judkins, multipurpose, left Amplatz, and pigtail

over three to five seconds by a motorised pump, providing visualisation of left ventricular contraction over two to four cardiac cycles. Aortic and ventricular pressures are also recorded during the procedure.

Intravascular ultrasound (IVUS)

In contrast to angiography, which gives a two dimensional luminal silhouette with little information about the vessel wall, intravascular ultrasound provides a cross sectional, three dimensional image of the full circumference of the artery. It allows precise measurement of plaque length and thickness and minimum lumen diameter, and it may also characterise the plaque's composition.

It is often used to clarify ambiguous angiographic findings and to identify wall dissections or thrombus. It is most useful during percutaneous coronary intervention, when target lesions can be assessed before, during, and after the procedure and at follow up. The procedure can also show that stents which seem to be well deployed on angiography are, in fact, suboptimally expanded. Its main limitations are the need for an operator experienced in its use and its expense; for these reasons it is not routinely used in many centres.

Doppler flow wire and pressure wire

Unlike angiography or intravascular ultrasound, the Doppler flow wire and pressure wire provide information on the physiological importance of a diseased coronary artery. They are usually used when angiography shows a stenosis that is of intermediate severity, or to determine the functional severity of a residual stenosis after percutaneous coronary intervention.

Intracoronary adenosine is used to dilate the distal coronary vessels in order to maximise coronary flow. The Doppler flow wire has a transducer at its tip, which is positioned beyond the stenosis to measure peak flow velocity. The pressure wire has a tip micrometer, which records arterial pressures proximal and distal to the stenosis.

The figure showing progression of atheromatous plaque from initial lesion is adapted with permission from Pepine CJ, *Am J Cardiol* 1998;82(suppl 10A):23-7S.

Competing interests: None declared.

Further reading

- Mark DB, Shaw L, Harrell FE Jr, Hlatky MA, Lee KL, Bengtson JR, et al. Prognostic value of a treadmill exercise score in outpatients with suspected coronary artery disease. *N Engl J Med* 1991;325: 849-53
- Marwick TH, Case C, Sawada S, Rimmerman C, Brenneman P, Kovacs R, et al. Prediction of mortality using dobutamine echocardiography. *J Am Coll Cardiol* 2001;37:754-60
- Scanlon PJ, Faxon DP, Audet AM, Carabello B, Dehmer GJ, Eagle KA, et al. ACC/AHA guidelines for coronary angiography. A report of the American College of Cardiology/American Heart Association Task Force on Practice Guidelines (Committee on Coronary Angiography). *J Am Coll Cardiol* 1999;33:1756-824
- Mintz GS, Nissen SE, Anderson WD, Bailey SR, Erbel R, Fitzgerald PJ, et al. American College of Cardiology clinical expert consensus document on standards for acquisition, measurement and reporting of intravascular ultrasound studies (IVUS). *J Am Coll Cardiol* 2001;37:1478-92

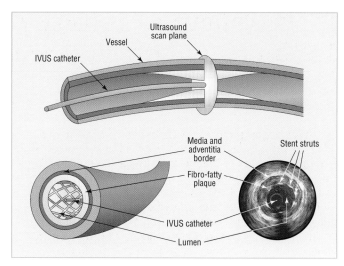

The intravascular ultrasound (IVUS) catheter (above) and images showing a stent within a diseased coronary artery (below)

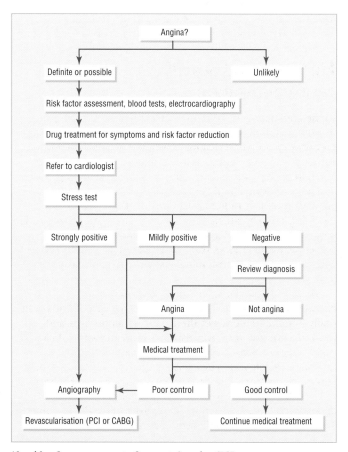

Algorithm for management of suspected angina (PCI=percutaneous coronary intervention, CABG=coronary artery bypass grafting)

2 Percutaneous coronary intervention. I: History and development

Ever D Grech

The term "angina pectoris" was introduced by Heberden in 1772 to describe a syndrome characterised by a sensation of "strangling and anxiety" in the chest. Today, it is used for chest discomfort attributed to myocardial ischaemia arising from increased myocardial oxygen consumption. This is often induced by physical exertion, and the commonest aetiology is atheromatous coronary artery disease. The terms "chronic" and "stable" refer to anginal symptoms that have been present for at least several weeks without major deterioration. However, symptom variation occurs for several reasons, such as mental stress, ambient temperature, consumption of alcohol or large meals, and factors that may increase coronary tone such as drugs and hormonal change.

Classification

The Canadian Cardiovascular Society has provided a graded classification of angina which has become widely used. In clinical practice, it is important to describe accurately specific activities associated with angina in each patient. This should include walking distance, frequency, and duration of episodes.

History of myocardial revascularisation

In the management of chronic stable angina, there are two invasive techniques available for myocardial revascularisation: coronary artery bypass surgery and catheter attached devices. Although coronary artery bypass surgery was introduced in 1968, the first percutaneous transluminal coronary angioplasty was not performed until September 1977 by Andreas Gruentzig, a Swiss radiologist, in Zurich. The patient, 38 year old Adolph Bachman, underwent successful angioplasty to a left coronary artery lesion and remains well to this day. After the success of the operation, six patients were successfully treated with percutaneous transluminal coronary angioplasty in that year.

By today's standards, the early procedures used cumbersome equipment: guide catheters were large and could easily traumatise the vessel, there were no guidewires, and balloon catheters were large with low burst pressures. As a result, the procedure was limited to patients with refractory angina, good left ventricular function, and a discrete, proximal, concentric, and non-calcific lesion in a single major coronary artery with no involvement of major side branches or angulations. Consequently, it was considered feasible in only 10% of all patients needing revascularisation.

Developments in percutaneous intervention

During 1977-86 guide catheters, guidewires, and balloon catheter technology were improved, with slimmer profiles and increased tolerance to high inflation pressures. As equipment improved and experience increased, so more complex lesions were treated and in more acute situations. Consequently,

Canadian Cardiovascular Society classification of angina

Class I
- No angina during ordinary physical activity such as walking or climbing stairs
- Angina during strenuous, rapid, or prolonged exertion

Class II
- Slight limitation of ordinary activity
- Angina on walking or climbing stairs rapidly; walking uphill; walking or climbing stairs shortly after meals, in cold or wind, when under emotional stress, or only in the first few hours after waking
- Angina on walking more than two blocks (100-200 m) on the level or climbing more than one flight of stairs at normal pace and in normal conditions

Class III
- Marked limitation of ordinary physical activity
- Angina on walking one or two blocks on the level or climbing one flight of stairs at normal pace and in normal conditions

Class IV
- Inability to carry out any physical activity without discomfort
- Includes angina at rest

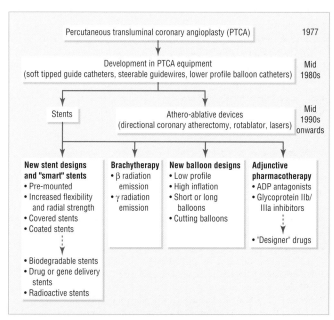

Major milestones in percutaneous coronary intervention

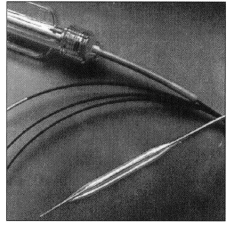

Modern balloon catheter: its low profile facilitates lesion crossing, the flexible shaft allows tracking down tortuous vessels, and the balloon can be inflated to high pressures without distortion or rupture

percutaneous transluminal coronary angioplasty can now be undertaken in about half of patients needing revascularisation (more in some countries), and it is also offered to high-risk patients for whom coronary artery bypass surgery may be considered too dangerous.

Although percutaneous transluminal coronary angioplasty causes plaque compression, the major change in lumen geometry is caused by fracturing and fissuring of the atheroma, extending into the vessel wall at variable depths and lengths. This injury accounts for the two major limitations of percutaneous transluminal coronary angioplasty-acute vessel closure and restenosis.

Acute vessel closure—This usually occurs within the first 24 hours of the procedure in about 3-5% of cases and follows vessel dissection, acute thrombus formation, or both. Important clinical consequences include myocardial infarction, emergency coronary artery bypass surgery, and death.

Restenosis occurring in the first six months after angioplasty is caused largely by smooth muscle cell proliferation and fibrointimal hyperplasia (often called neointimal proliferation), as well as elastic recoil. It is usually defined as a greater than 50% reduction in luminal diameter and has an incidence of 25-50% (higher after vein graft angioplasty). Further intervention may be indicated if angina and ischaemia recur.

Drills, cutters, and lasers

In the 1980s, two main developments aimed at limiting these problems emerged. The first were devices to remove plaque material, such as by rotational atherectomy, directional coronary atherectomy, transluminal extraction catheter, and excimer laser. By avoiding the vessel wall trauma seen during percutaneous transluminal coronary angioplasty, it was envisaged that both acute vessel closure and restenosis rates would be reduced.

However, early studies showed that, although acute closure rates were reduced, there was no significant reduction in restenosis. Moreover, these devices are expensive, not particularly user friendly, and have limited accessibility to more distal stenoses. As a result, they have now become niche tools used by relatively few interventionists. However, they may have an emerging role in reducing restenosis rates when used as adjunctive treatment before stenting (especially for large plaques) and in treating diffuse restenosis within a stent.

Intracoronary stents

The second development was the introduction of intracoronary stents deployed at the site of an atheromatous lesion. These were introduced in 1986 with the objective of tacking down dissection flaps and providing mechanical support. They also reduce elastic recoil and remodelling associated with restenosis.

The first large randomised studies conclusively showed the superiority of stenting over coronary angioplasty alone, both in clinical and angiographic outcomes, including a significant 30% reduction in restenosis rates. Surprisingly, this was not due to inhibition of neointimal proliferation—in fact stents may increase this response. The superiority of stenting is that the initial gain in luminal diameter is much greater than after angioplasty alone, mostly because of a reduction in elastic recoil.

Although neointimal proliferation through the struts of the stent occurs, it is insufficient to cancel out the initial gain, leading to a larger lumen size and hence reduced restenosis. Maximising the vessel lumen is therefore a crucial mechanism for reducing restenosis. "Bigger is better" is the adage followed in this case.

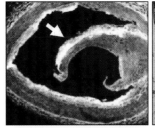
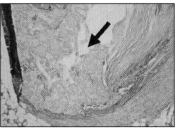
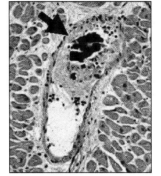

Micrographs showing arterial barotrauma caused by coronary angioplasty. Top left: coronary arterial dissection with large flap. Top right: deep fissuring within coronary artery wall atheroma. Bottom: fragmented plaque tissue (dark central calcific plaque surrounded by fibrin and platelet-rich thrombus), which may embolise in distal arterioles to cause infarction

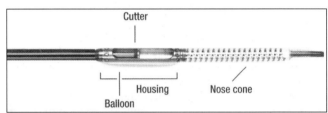

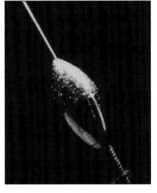

Tools for coronary atherectomy. Top: the Simpson atherocath has a cutter in a hollow cylindrical housing. The cutter rotates at 2000 rpm, and excised atheromatous tissue is pushed into the distal nose cone. Left: the Rotablator burr is coated with 10 µm diamond chips to create an abrasive surface. The burr, connected to a drive shaft and a turbine powered by compressed air, rotates at speeds up to 200 000 rpm

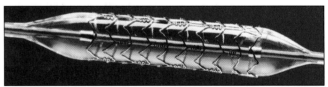
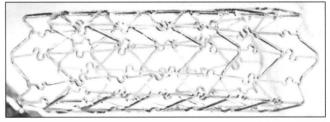
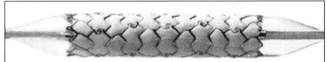

Coronary stents. Top: Guidant Zeta stent. Middle: BiodivYsio AS stent coated with phosphorylcholine, a synthetic copy of the outer membrane of red blood cells, which improves haemocompatibility and reduces thrombosis. Bottom: the Jomed JOSTENT coronary stent graft consists of a layer of PTFE (polytetrafluoroethylene) sandwiched between two stents and is useful in sealing perforations, aneurysms, and fistulae

Early stent problems

As a result of initial studies, stents were predominantly used either as "bail out" devices for acute vessel closure during coronary angioplasty (thus avoiding the need for immediate coronary artery bypass surgery) or for restenosis after angioplasty.

Thrombosis within a stent causing myocardial infarction and death was a major concern, and early aggressive anticoagulation to prevent this led to frequent complications from arterial puncture wounds as well as major systemic haemorrhage. These problems have now been overcome by the introduction of powerful antiplatelet drugs as a substitute for warfarin. The risk of thrombosis within a stent diminishes when the stent is lined with a new endothelial layer, and antiplatelet treatment can be stopped after a month. The recognition that suboptimal stent expansion is an important contributor to thrombosis in stents has led to the use of intravascular ultrasound to guide stent deployment and high pressure inflations to ensure complete stent expansion.

Current practice

A greater understanding of the pathophysiology of stent deployment, combined with the development of more flexible stents (which are pre-mounted on low-profile catheter balloons), has resulted in a massive worldwide increase in stent use, and they have become an essential component of coronary intervention. Low profile stents have also allowed "direct" stenting—that is, implanting a stent without the customary balloon dilatation—to become prevalent, with the advantages of economy, shorter procedure time, and less radiation from imaging. Most modern stents are expanded by balloon and made from stainless steel alloys. Their construction and design, metal thickness, surface coverage, and radial strength vary considerably.

Stents are now used in most coronary interventions and in a wide variety of clinical settings. They substantially increase procedural safety and success, and reduce the need for emergency coronary artery bypass surgery. Procedures involving stent deployment are now often referred to as percutaneous coronary interventions to distinguish them from conventional balloon angioplasty (percutaneous transluminal coronary angioplasty).

A major recent development has been the introduction of drug eluting stents (also referred to as "coated stents"), which reduce restenosis to very low rates. Their high cost currently limits their use, but, with increasing competition among manufacturers, they will probably become more affordable.

Competing interests: None declared.

The micrographs showing deep fissuring within a coronary artery wall atheroma and fragmented plaque tissue caused by coronary angioplasty were supplied by Kelly MacDonald, consultant histopathologist at St Boniface Hospital, Winnipeg, Canada.

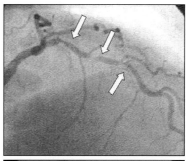
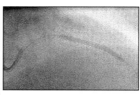
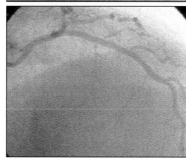

Coronary angiogram showing three lesions (arrows) affecting the left anterior descending artery (top left). The lesions are stented without pre-dilatation (top right), with good results (bottom)

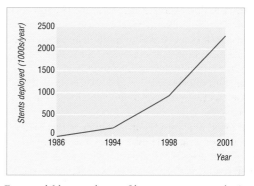

Exponential increase in use of intracoronary stents since 1986. In 2001, 2.3 million stents were implanted (more than double the 1998 rate)

Unequivocal indications for use of coronary stents

- Acute or threatened vessel closure during angioplasty
- Primary reduction in restenosis in de novo lesions in arteries >3.0 mm in diameter
- Focal lesions in saphenous vein grafts
- Recanalised total chronic occlusions
- Primary treatment of acute coronary syndromes

Further reading

- Gruentzig AR. Transluminal dilatation of coronary artery stenosis. *Lancet* 1978;1:263
- Smith SC Jr, Dove JT, Jacobs AK, Kennedy JW, Kereiakes D, Kern MJ, et al. ACC/AHA guidelines of percutaneous coronary interventions (revision of the 1993 PTCA guidelines)—executive summary. A report of the American College of Cardiology/ American Heart Association Task Force on Practice Guidelines (committee to revise the 1993 guidelines for percutaneous transluminal coronary angioplasty). *J Am Coll Cardiol* 2001;37: 2215-39
- Meyer BJ, Meier B. Percutaneous transluminal coronary angioplasty of single or multivessel disease and chronic total occlusions. In: Grech ED, Ramsdale DR, eds. *Practical interventional cardiology*. 2nd ed. London: Martin Dunitz, 2002:35-54
- Costa MA, Foley DP, Serruys PW. Restenosis: the problem and how to deal with it. In: Grech ED, Ramsdale DR, eds. *Practical interventional cardiology*. 2nd ed. London: Martin Dunitz, 2002: 279-94
- Topol EJ, Serruys PW. Frontiers in interventional cardiology. *Circulation* 1998;98:1802-20

3 Percutaneous coronary intervention.
II: The procedure

Ever D Grech

A wide range of patients may be considered for percutaneous coronary intervention. It is essential that the benefits and risks of the procedure, as well as coronary artery bypass graft surgery and medical treatment, are discussed with patients (and their families) in detail. They must understand that, although the percutaneous procedure is more attractive than bypass surgery, it has important limitations, including the likelihood of restenosis and potential for incomplete revascularisation compared with surgery. The potential benefits of antianginal drug treatment and the need for risk factor reduction should also be carefully explained.

Clinical risk assessment

Relief of anginal symptoms is the principal clinical indication for percutaneous intervention, but we do not know whether the procedure has the same prognostic benefit as bypass surgery. Angiographic features determined during initial assessment require careful evaluation to determine the likely success of the procedure and the risk of serious complications.

Until recently, the American College of Cardiology and American Heart Association classified anginal lesions into types (and subtypes) A, B, or C based on the severity of lesion characteristics. Because of the ability of stents to overcome many of the complications of percutaneous intervention, this classification has now been superseded by one reflecting low, moderate, and high risk.

Successful percutaneous intervention depends on adequate visualisation of the target stenosis and its adjacent arterial branches. Vessels beyond the stenosis may also be important because of the potential for collateral flow and myocardial support if the target vessel were to occlude abruptly. Factors that adversely affect outcome include increasing age, comorbid disease, unstable angina, pre-existing heart or renal failure, previous myocardial infarction, diabetes, a large area of myocardium at risk, degree of collaterisation, and multivessel disease.

Preparation for intervention

Patients must be fully informed of the purpose of the procedure as well as its risks and limitations before they are asked for their consent. The procedure must always be carried out (or directly supervised) by experienced, high volume operators (>75 procedures a year) and institutions (>400 a year).

A sedative is often given before the procedure, as well as aspirin, clopidogrel, and the patient's usual antianginal drugs. In very high risk cases an intra-aortic balloon pump may be used. A prophylactic temporary transvenous pacemaker wire may be inserted in some patients with pre-existing, high grade conduction abnormality or those at high risk of developing it.

The procedure

For an uncomplicated, single lesion, a percutaneous procedure may take as little as 30 minutes. However, the duration of the procedure and radiation exposure will vary according to thenumber and complexity of the treated stenoses and vessels.

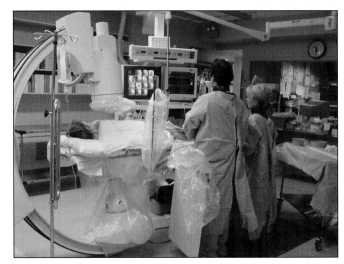

Percutaneous coronary intervention in progress. Above the patient's chest is the x ray imaging camera. Fluoroscopic images, electrocardiogram, and haemodynamic data are viewed at eye level screens. All catheterisation laboratory operators wear lead protection covering body, thyroid, and eyes, and there is lead shielding between the primary operator and patient

New classification system of stenotic lesions (American College of Cardiology and American Heart Association)

Low risk	Moderate risk	High risk
Discrete (<10 mm)	Tubular (10-20 mm)	Diffuse (>20 mm)
Concentric	Eccentric	
Readily accessible	Proximal segment moderately tortuous	Proximal segment excessively tortuous
Segment not angular (<45°)	Segment moderately angular (45°-<90°)	Segment extremely angular (≥90°)
Smooth contour	Irregular contour	
Little or no calcification	Moderate or heavy calcification	
Occlusion not total	Total occlusion <3 months old	Total occlusion >3 months or bridging collateral vessels
Non-ostial	Ostial	
No major side branch affected	Bifurcated lesions requiring double guidewires	Inability to protect major side branches
No thrombus	Some thrombus	Degenerated vein grafts with friable lesions.

Clinical indications for percutaneous coronary intervention

- Stable angina (and positive stress test)
- Unstable angina
- Acute myocardial infarction
- After myocardial infarction
- After coronary artery bypass surgery (percutaneous intervention to native vessels, arterial or venous conduits)
- High risk bypass surgery
- Elderly patient

As with coronary angiography, arterial access (usually femoral but also brachial or radial) under local anaesthesia is required. A guide catheter is introduced and gently engaged at the origin of the coronary artery. The proximal end of the catheter is attached to a Y connector. One arm of this connector allows continuous monitoring of arterial blood pressure. Dampening or "ventricularisation" of this arterial tracing may indicate reduced coronary flow because of over-engagement of the guide catheter, catheter tip spasm, or a previously unrecognised ostial lesion. The other arm has an adjustable seal, through which the operator can introduce the guidewire and balloon or stent catheter once the patient has been given heparin as an anticoagulant. A glycoprotein IIb/IIIa inhibitor, which substantially reduces ischaemic events during percutaneous coronary intervention, may also be given.

Visualised by means of fluoroscopy and intracoronary injections of contrast medium, a soft tipped, steerable guidewire (usually 0.014" (0.36 mm) diameter) is passed down the coronary artery, across the stenosis, and into a distal branch. A balloon or stent catheter is then passed over the guidewire and positioned at the stenosis. The stenosis may then be stented directly or dilated before stenting. Additional balloon dilatation may be necessary after deployment of a stent to ensure its full expansion.

Balloon inflation inevitably stops coronary blood flow, which may induce angina. Patients usually tolerate this quite well, especially if they have been warned beforehand. If it becomes severe or prolonged, however, an intravenous opiate may be given. Ischaemic electrocardiographic changes are often seen at this time, although they are usually transient and return to baseline once the balloon is deflated (usually after 30-60 seconds). During the procedure, it is important to talk to the patient (who may be understandably apprehensive) to let him or her know what is happening, as this encourages a good rapport and cooperation.

Recovery

After the procedure the patient is transferred to a ward where close monitoring for signs of ischaemia and haemodynamic instability is available. If a femoral arterial sheath was used, it may be removed when the heparin effect has declined to an acceptable level (according to unit protocols). Arterial sealing devices have some advantages over manual compression: they permit immediate sheath removal and haemostasis, are more comfortable for patients, and allow early mobilisation and discharge. However, they are not widely used as they add considerably to the cost of the procedure.

After a few hours, the patient should be encouraged to gradually increase mobility, and in uncomplicated cases discharge is scheduled for the same or the next day. Before discharge, the arterial access site should be examined and the patient advised to seek immediate medical advice if bleeding or chest pain (particularly at rest) occurs. Outpatient follow up and drug regimens are provided, as well as advice on modification of risk factors and lifestyle.

Complications and sequelae

Complications are substantially lower in centres where large numbers of procedures are carried out by adequately trained and experienced operators. Major complications are uncommon and include death (0.2% but higher in high risk cases), acute myocardial infarction (1%) which may require emergency coronary artery bypass surgery, embolic stroke (0.5%), cardiac tamponade (0.5%), and systemic bleeding (0.5%).

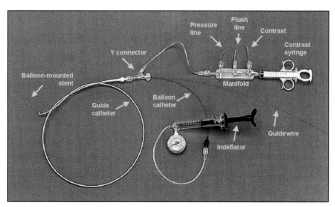

Equipment commonly used in percutaneous coronary interventions

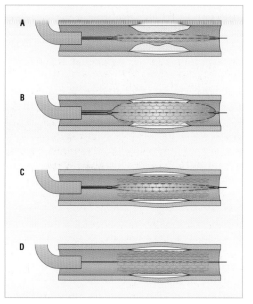

Deployment of a balloon-mounted stent across stenotic lesion. Once the guide catheter is satisfactorily engaged, the lesion is crossed with a guidewire and the balloon-mounted stent positioned to cover the lesion (A). It may be necessary to pre-dilate a severe lesion with a balloon to provide adequate passageway for the balloon and stent. The balloon is inflated to expand the stent (B). The balloon is then deflated (C) and withdrawn leaving the guidewire (D), which is also removed once the operator is satisfied that a good result has been obtained

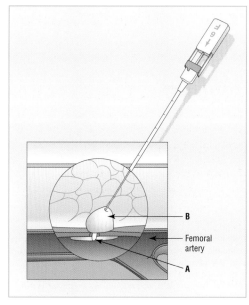

Example of a femoral artery closure device. The Angio-Seal device creates a mechanical seal by sandwiching the arteriotomy between an anchor placed against the inner arterial wall (A) and collagen sponge (B), which both dissolve within 60-90 days

ABC of Interventional Cardiology

Minor complications are more common and include allergy to the contrast medium and nephropathy and complications of the access site (bleeding, haematoma, and pseudoaneurysm).

Restenosis within a stent

Although stents prevent restenosis from vascular recoil and remodelling, restenosis within the stent (known as "in-stent restenosis") due to neointimal proliferation does occur and is the most important late sequel of the procedure. In-stent restenosis is the Achilles' heel of percutaneous revascularisation and develops within six months of stenting.

Angiographic restenosis rates ($>50\%$ diameter stenosis) depend on several factors and are higher in smaller vessels, long and complex stenoses, and where there are coexisting conditions such as diabetes. Approximate rates of angiographic restenosis after percutaneous angioplasty are

- Angioplasty to de novo lesion in native artery—35%
- Angioplasty and stent to de novo lesion in native artery—25%
- Angioplasty and stent to restenotic lesion in native artery—20%
- Angioplasty and stent to successfully recanalised chronic total occlusion—30%
- Angioplasty to de novo lesion in vein graft—60%
- Angioplasty and stent to de novo lesion in vein graft—30%.

It should be noted that angiographically apparent restenoses do not always lead to recurrent angina (clinical restenosis). In some patients only mild anginal symptoms recur, and these may be well controlled with antianginal drugs, thereby avoiding the need for further intervention.

Using repeat percutaneous angioplasty alone to re-dilate in-stent restenosis results in a high recurrence of restenosis (60%). Various other methods, such as removing restenotic tissue by means of atherectomy or a laser device or re-dilating with a cutting balloon, are being evaluated. Another method is brachytherapy, which uses a special intracoronary catheter to deliver a source of β or γ radiation. It significantly reduces further in-stent restenosis, but it has limitations, including late thrombosis and new restenosis at the edges of the radiation treated segments, giving rise to a "candy wrapper" appearance.

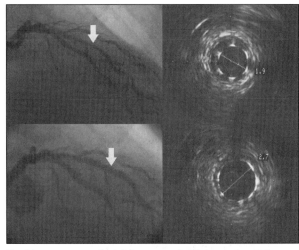

Focal in-stent restenosis. A 2.0 mm stent had been deployed six months earlier. After recurrence of angina, angiography showed focal in-stent restenosis (arrow, top left). This was confirmed with intravascular ultrasound (top right), which also revealed that the stent was underexpanded. The stent was further expanded with a balloon catheter, with a good angiographic result (arrow, bottom left) and an increased lumen diameter to 2.7 mm (bottom right)

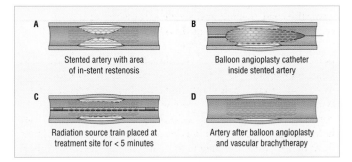

Diagrammatic representation of the Novoste Beta Cath system used for vascular brachytherapy. Pre-dilatation of the in-stent restenosis with a balloon catheter is usual and is followed by positioning of the radiation source train, containing strontium-90, at the site for less than 5 minutes

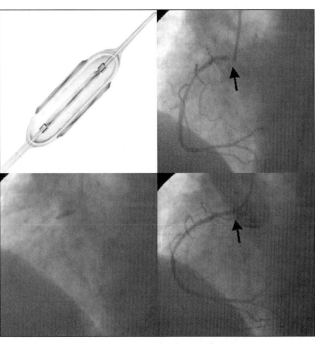

The cutting balloon catheter. The longitudinal cutting blades are exposed only during balloon inflation (top left). In this case (top right) a severe ostial in-stent restenosis in the right coronary artery (arrow) was dilated with a short cutting balloon (bottom left), and a good angiographic result was obtained (arrow, bottom right)

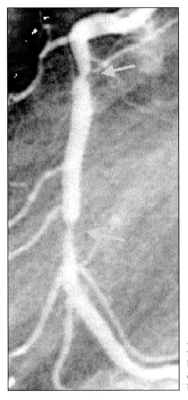

Angiogram showing late "candy wrapper" edge effect (arrows) because of new restenosis at the edges of a segment treated by brachytherapy

Drug eluting, coated stents

Coated stents contain drugs that inhibit new tissue growth within the sub-intima and are a promising new option for preventing or treating in-stent restenosis. Sirolimus (an immunosuppressant used to prevent renal rejection which inhibits smooth muscle proliferation and reduces intimal thickening after vascular injury), paclitaxel (the active component of the anticancer drug taxol), everolimus, ABT-578, and tacrolimus are all being studied, as are other agents. Although long term data and cost benefit analyses are not yet available, it seems probable that coated stents will be commonly used in the near future.

Occupation and driving

Doctors may be asked to advise on whether a patient is "fit for work" or "recovered from an event" after percutaneous coronary intervention. "Fitness" depends on clinical factors (level of symptoms, extent and severity of coronary disease, left ventricular function, stress test result) and the nature of the occupation, as well as statutory and non-statutory fitness requirements. Advisory medical standards are in place for certain occupations, such as in the armed forces and police, railwaymen, and professional divers. Statutory requirements cover the road, marine, and aviation industries and some recreational pursuits such as driving and flying.

Patients often ask when they may resume driving after percutaneous coronary intervention. In Britain, the Driver and Vehicle Licensing Agency recommends that group 1 (private motor car) licence holders should stop driving when anginal symptoms occur at rest or at the wheel. After percutaneous coronary intervention, they should not drive for a week. Drivers holding a group 2 licence (lorries or buses) will be disqualified from driving once the diagnosis of angina has been made, and for at least six weeks after percutaneous coronary intervention. Re-licensing may be permitted provided the exercise test requirement (satisfactory completion of nine minutes of the Bruce protocol while not taking β blockers) can be met and there is no other disqualifying condition.

The diagram of the Angio-Seal device is used with permission of St Jude Medical, Minnetonka, Minnesota, USA. The angiogram showing the "candy wrapper" effect is reproduced with permission of R Waksman, Washington Hospital Center, and Martin Dunitz, London.

Competing interests: None declared.

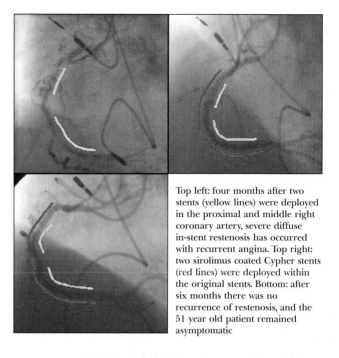

Top left: four months after two stents (yellow lines) were deployed in the proximal and middle right coronary artery, severe diffuse in-stent restenosis has occurred with recurrent angina. Top right: two sirolimus coated Cypher stents (red lines) were deployed within the original stents. Bottom: after six months there was no recurrence of restenosis, and the 51 year old patient remained asymptomatic

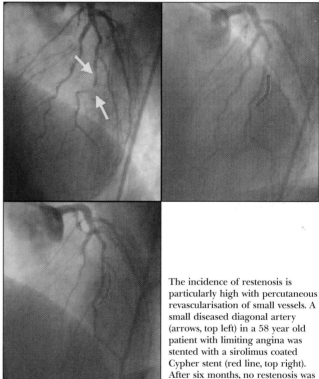

The incidence of restenosis is particularly high with percutaneous revascularisation of small vessels. A small diseased diagonal artery (arrows, top left) in a 58 year old patient with limiting angina was stented with a sirolimus coated Cypher stent (red line, top right). After six months, no restenosis was present (left), and the patient remained asymptomatic

Further reading

- Smith SC Jr, Dove JT, Jacobs AK, Kennedy JW, Kereiakes D, Kern MJ, et al. ACC/AHA guidelines of percutaneous coronary interventions (revision of the 1993 PTCA guidelines)—executive summary. A report of the American College of Cardiology/ American Heart Association Task Force on Practice Guidelines (committee to revise the 1993 guidelines for percutaneous transluminal coronary angioplasty). *J Am Coll Cardiol* 2001;37: 2215-39
- Morice MC, Serruys PW, Sousa JE, Fajadet J, Ban Hayashi E, Perin M, et al. A randomized comparison of a sirolimus-eluting stent with a standard stent for coronary revascularization. *N Engl J Med* 2002;346:1773-80
- Almond DG. Coronary stenting I: intracoronary stents—form, function future. In: Grech ED, Ramsdale DR, eds. *Practical interventional cardiology*. 2nd ed. London: Martin Dunitz, 2002:63-76
- Waksman R. Management of restenosis through radiation therapy. In: Grech ED, Ramsdale DR, eds. *Practical interventional cardiology*. 2nd ed. London: Martin Dunitz, 2002:295-305
- Kimmel SE, Berlin JA, Laskey WK. The relationship between coronary angioplasty procedure volume and major complications. *JAMA* 1995;274:1137-42
- Rensing BJ, Vos J, Smits PC, Foley DP, van den Brand MJ, van der Giessen WJ, et al. Coronary restenosis elimination with a sirolimus eluting stent. *Eur Heart J* 2001;22:2125-30

4 Chronic stable angina: treatment options

Laurence O'Toole, Ever D Grech

In patients with chronic stable angina, the factors influencing the choice of coronary revascularisation therapy (percutaneous coronary intervention or coronary artery bypass surgery) are varied and complex. The severity of symptoms, lifestyle, extent of objective ischaemia, and underlying risks must be weighed against the benefits of revascularisation and the patient's preference, as well as local availability and expertise. Evidence from randomised trials and large revascularisation registers can guide these decisions, but the past decade has seen rapid change in medical treatment, bypass surgery, and percutaneous intervention. Therefore, thought must be given to whether older data still apply to contemporary practice.

Patients with chronic stable angina have an average annual mortality of 2-3%, only twice that of age matched controls, and this relatively benign prognosis is an important consideration when determining the merits of revascularisation treatment. Certain patients, however, are at much higher risk. Predictors include poor exercise capacity with easily inducible ischaemia or a poor haemodynamic response to exercise, angina of recent onset, previous myocardial infarction, impaired left ventricular function, and the number of coronary vessels with significant stenoses, especially when disease affects the left main stem or proximal left anterior descending artery. Although the potential benefits of revascularisation must be weighed against adverse factors, those most at risk may have the most to gain.

Treatment strategies

Medical treatment
Anti-ischaemic drugs improve symptoms and quality of life, but have not been shown to reduce mortality or myocardial infarction. β blockers may improve survival in hypertension, in heart failure, and after myocardial infarction, and so are considered by many to be first line treatment. Nicorandil has recently been shown to reduce ischaemic events and need for hospital admission.

Trials comparing medical treatment with revascularisation predate the widespread use of antiplatelet and cholesterol lowering drugs. These drugs reduce risk, both in patients treated with drugs only and in those undergoing revascularisation, and so may have altered the risk-benefit ratio for a particular revascularisation strategy in some patients.

Coronary artery bypass graft surgery
Coronary artery bypass surgery involves the placement of grafts to bypass stenosed native coronary arteries, while maintaining cerebral and peripheral circulation by cardiopulmonary bypass. The grafts are usually saphenous veins or arteries (principally the left internal mammary artery).

Operative mortality is generally 1-3% but may be much higher in certain subsets of patients. Scoring systems can predict operative mortality based on clinical, investigational, and operative factors. Important developments that have occurred since trials of bypass surgery versus medical treatment were conducted include increased use of arterial grafts (which have much greater longevity than venous grafts), surgery without extracorporeal circulation ("off-pump" bypass), and minimal access surgery.

Major factors influencing risks and benefits of coronary revascularisation

- Advanced age
- Female
- Severe angina
- Smoking
- Diabetes
- Obesity
- Hypertension

- Multiple coronary vessels affected
- Coexisting valve disease
- Impaired left ventricular function
- Impaired renal function
- Cerebrovascular or peripheral vascular disease
- Recent acute coronary syndrome
- Chronic obstructive airways disease

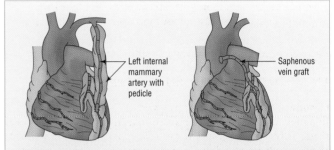

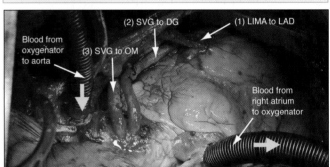

Top: Diagrams of saphenous vein and left internal mammary artery grafts for coronary artery bypass surgery. Bottom: Three completed grafts—(1) left internal mammary artery (LIMA) to left anterior descending artery (LAD), and saphenous vein grafts (SVG) to (2) diagonal artery (DG) and (3) obtuse marginal artery (OM)

Risk score for assessing probable mortality from bypass surgery in patients with chronic stable angina

Risk factor	Weighted score
Age >60	Score 1 for every 5 years over
Female sex	1
Chronic obstructive pulmonary disease	1
Extracardiac arteriopathy	2
Neurological dysfunction	2
Previous cardiac surgery	3
Serum creatinine >200µmol/l	2
Reduced left ventricular ejection fraction	1 for 30-50% 3 for <30%
Myocardial infarction in past 90 days	2
Pulmonary artery systolic pressure >60 mm Hg	2
Major cardiac procedure as well as bypass surgery	2
Emergency operation	2

- Total score ≤2 predicts <1% operative mortality
- Total score of 3-5 predicts 3% operative mortality
- Total score ≥6 predicts >10% operative mortality

A more detailed assessment with logistic analysis is available at www.euroscore.org and is recommended for assessing high risk patients

Percutaneous coronary intervention

The main advantages of percutaneous intervention over bypass surgery are the avoidance of the risks of general anaesthesia, uncomfortable sternotomy and saphenous wounds, and complications of major surgery (infections and pulmonary emboli). Only an overnight hospital stay is necessary (and many procedures can be performed as day cases), and the procedure can be easily repeated. The mortality is low (0.2%), and the most serious late complication is restenosis.

Patient suitability is primarily determined by technical factors. A focal stenosis on a straight artery without proximal vessel tortuousness or involvement of major side branches is ideal for percutaneous intervention. Long, heavily calcified stenoses in tortuous vessels or at bifurcations and chronic total occlusions are less suitable. This must be borne in mind when interpreting data from trials of percutaneous intervention and bypass surgery, as only a minority of patients were suitable for both procedures. Nowadays, more and more patients undergo percutaneous intervention, and referral rates for bypass surgery are falling.

Comparative studies of revascularisation strategies

Coronary artery bypass surgery versus medical treatment

In a meta-analysis of seven trials comparing bypass surgery with medical treatment, surgery conferred a survival advantage in patients with severe left main stem coronary disease, three vessel disease, or two vessel disease with severely affected proximal left anterior descending artery. The survival gain was more pronounced in patients with left ventricular dysfunction or a strongly positive exercise test. However, only 10% of trial patients received an internal mammary artery graft, only 25% received antiplatelet drugs, and the benefit of lipid lowering drugs on long term graft patency was not appreciated when these studies were carried out. Furthermore, 40% of the medically treated patients underwent bypass surgery during 10 years of follow up. Thus, these data may underestimate the benefits of surgery compared with medical treatment alone.

In lower risk patients bypass surgery is indicated only for symptom relief and to improve quality of life when medical treatment has failed. Surgery does this effectively, with 95% of patients gaining immediate relief from angina and 75% remaining free from angina after five years. Unfortunately, venous grafts have a median life span of only seven years, and after 15 years only 15% of patients are free from recurrent angina or death or myocardial infarction. However, the increased use of internal mammary artery grafts, which have excellent long term patency (85% at 10 years), has increased postoperative survival and reduced long term symptoms.

Subgroup analysis of mortality benefit from coronary artery bypass surgery compared with medical treatment at 10 years after randomisation for patients with chronic stable angina

Subgroup	Mean (1.96 SE) increased survival time (months)	P value of difference
Vessel disease:		
1 or 2 vessels	1.8 (3.0)	0.25
3 vessels	5.7 (3.6)	0.001
Left main stem	19.3 (13.7)	0.005
Left ventricular function:		
Normal	2.3 (2.4)	0.06
Abnormal	10.6 (6.1)	<0.001
Exercise test:		
Normal	3.3 (4.4)	0.14
Abnormal	5.1 (3.3)	0.002
Severity of angina:		
CCS class 0, I, II	3.3 (2.7)	0.02
CCS class III, IV	7.3 (4.8)	0.002

CCS=Canadian Cardiovascular Society

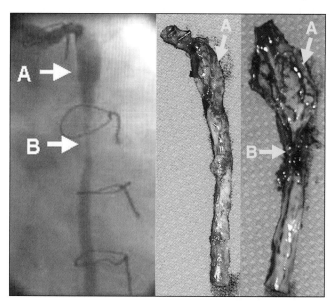

Left: Angiogram of a 10 year old diseased venous graft to the obtuse marginal artery showing proximal aneurysmal dilatation (A) and severe stenosis in middle segment (B). Right: Removal of this graft after repeat bypass surgery shows its gross appearance (graft longitudinally opened in right image), with atherosclerosis in a thin walled aneurysm and a small residual lumen

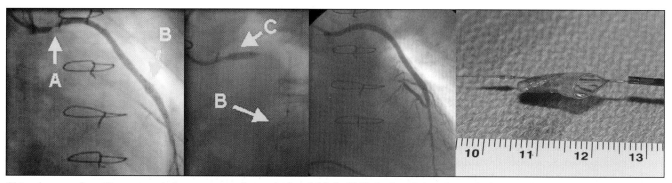

Old saphenous vein grafts may contain large amounts of necrotic clotted debris, friable laminated thrombus, and ulcerated atheromatous plaque and are unattractive for percutaneous intervention because of the high risk of distal embolisation. However, distal embolisation protection devices such as the FilterWire EX (far right) reduce this risk by trapping any material released. Such a device (far left, B) is positioned in the distal segment of a subtotally occluded saphenous vein graft of the left anterior descending artery (A) before it is dilated and stented (inner left, C) to restore blood flow (inner right)

Percutaneous coronary intervention versus medical treatment

Most percutaneous procedures are undertaken to treat single vessel or two vessel disease, but few randomised controlled trials have compared percutaneous intervention with medical treatment. These showed that patients undergoing the percutaneous procedure derived greater angina relief and took less drugs but required more subsequent procedures and had more complications (including non-fatal myocardial infarction), with no mortality difference. Patients with few symptoms did not derive benefit. Therefore, percutaneous intervention is suitable for low risk patients with one or two vessel disease and poor symptom control with drugs, at a cost of a slightly higher risk of non-fatal myocardial infarction. However, the procedure may not be indicated if symptoms are well controlled.

Percutaneous intervention versus bypass surgery

Single vessel disease

In a meta-analysis by Pocock et al percutaneous intervention in patients with single vessel disease resulted in mortality similar to that found with bypass surgery (3.7% v 3.1% respectively) but a higher rate of non-fatal myocardial infarction (10.1% v 6.1%, P=0.04). Angina was well treated in both groups, but persistence of symptoms was slightly higher with percutaneous intervention. Rates of repeat rcvascularisation wcrc much higher with percutaneous intervention than bypass surgery.

Multivessel disease

Since comparative trials could recruit only those patients who were suitable for either revascularisation strategy, only 3-7% of screened patients were included. These were predominantly "low risk" patients with two vessel disease and preserved left ventricular function—patients in whom bypass surgery has not been shown to improve survival—and thus it is unlikely that a positive effect in favour of percutaneous intervention would have been detected. The generally benign prognosis of chronic stable angina means that much larger trials would have been required to show significant differences in mortality.

A meta-analysis of data available to the end of 2000 revealed similar rates of death and myocardial infarction with both procedures, but repeat revascularisation rates were higher with percutaneous intervention. The prevalence of appreciable angina was greater with percutaneous intervention at one year, but this difference disappeared at three years.

The nature of percutaneous coronary intervention has changed considerably over the past 10 years, with important developments including stenting and improved antiplatelet drugs. The integrated use of these treatments clearly improves outcomes, but almost all of the revascularisation trials predate these developments.

A more recent trial comparing percutaneous intervention and stenting with bypass surgery in multivessel disease confirmed similar rates of death, myocardial infarction, and stroke at one year, with much lower rates of repeat revascularisation after percutaneous intervention compared with earlier trials. There was also a cost benefit of nearly $3000 (£1875) per patient associated with percutaneous intervention at 12 months. The recent introduction of drug eluting (coated) stents, which seem to reduce substantially the problem of restenosis, is likely to extend the use of percutaneous intervention in multivessel disease over the next few years.

Diabetes

Bypass surgery confers a survival advantage in symptomatic diabetic patients with multivessel disease The BARI trial

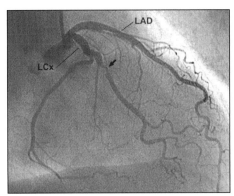

Coronary angiogram showing a severe focal stenosis (arrow) in a large oblique marginal branch of the left circumflex artery (LCx), suitable for percutaneous coronary intervention. The left anterior descending artery (LAD) has no important disease

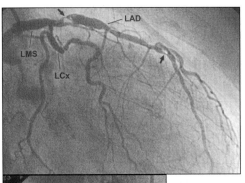

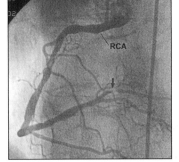

Coronary angiograms of 70 year old woman with limiting angina. There were severe stenoses (arrows) in the proximal and middle left anterior descending artery (LAD, top) and in the distal right coronary artery (RCA, left). Because of the focal nature of these lesions, percutaneous coronary intervention was the preferred option

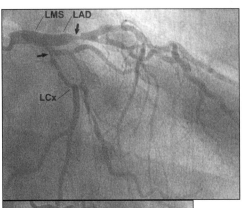

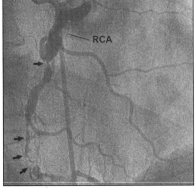

Coronary angiograms of a 69 year old man with limiting angina and exertional breathlessness. There was severe proximal disease (arrows) of the left anterior descending (LAD) and left circumflex arteries (LCx) (top) and occlusion of the right coronary artery (RCA, left). The patient was referred for coronary artery bypass surgery on prognostic and symptomatic grounds

revealed a significant difference in five year mortality (21% with percutaneous intervention *v* 6% with bypass surgery). Similar trends have been found in other large trials. However, the recent RAVEL and SIRIUS studies, in which the sirolimus eluting Cypher stent was compared with the same stent uncoated, showed a remarkable reduction in restenosis rates within the stented segments in diabetic patients (0% *v* 42% and 18% *v* 51% respectively). Ongoing trials will investigate this issue further.

Other study data

Large registries of outcomes in patients undergoing revascularisation have the advantage of including all patients rather than the highly selected groups included in randomised trials. The registry data seem to agree with those from randomised trials: patients with more extensive disease fare better with bypass surgery, whereas percutaneous intervention is preferable in focal coronary artery disease.

An unusual observation is that patients screened and considered suitable for inclusion in a trial fared slightly better if they refused to participate than did those who enrolled. The heterogeneous nature of coronary disease means that certain patient subsets will probably benefit more from one treatment than another. The better outcome in the patients who were suitable but not randomised may indicate that cardiologists and surgeons recognise which patients will benefit more from a particular strategy—subtleties that are lost in the randomisation process of controlled trials.

Refractory coronary artery disease

Increasing numbers of patients with coronary artery disease have angina that is unresponsive to both maximal drug treatment and revascularisation techniques. Many will have already undergone multiple percutaneous interventions or bypass surgery procedures, or have diffuse and distal coronary artery disease. In addition to functional limitations, their prognosis may be poor because of impaired ventricular function. Emerging treatments may provide alternative symptomatic improvement for some patients. There is also renewed interest in the potential anti-ischaemic effects of angiotensin converting enzyme inhibitors and the plaque stabilising properties of statins.

The picture showing three completed coronary artery bypass grafts and the pictures of a 10 year old diseased venous graft to the obtuse marginal artery were provided by G Singh, consultant cardiothoracic surgeon, Heath Sciences Centre, Winnipeg, E Pascoe, consultant cardiothoracic surgeon, St Boniface Hospital, Winnipeg, and J Scatliff, consultant anaesthetist, St Boniface Hospital. The picture of the FilterWire EX distal embolisation protection device was provided by Boston Scientific Corporation, Minneapolis, USA.

Competing interests: None declared.

Emerging treatment options for refractory angina
- *Drugs*—Analgesics, statins, angiotensin converting enzyme inhibitors, antiplatelet drugs
- *Neurostimulation*—Interruption or modification of afferent nociceptive signals: transcutaneous electric nerve stimulation (TENS), spinal cord stimulation (SCS)
- *Enhanced external counterpulsation*—Non-invasive pneumatic leg compression, improving coronary perfusion and decreasing left ventricular afterload
- *Laser revascularisation*—Small myocardial channels created by laser beams: transmyocardial laser revascularisation (TMLR), percutaneous transmyocardial laser revascularisation (PTMLR)
- *Therapeutic angiogenesis*—Cytokines, vascular endothelial growth factor, and fibroblast growth factor injected into ischaemic myocardium, or adenoviral vector for gene transport to promote neovascularisation
- *Percutaneous in situ coronary venous arterialisation (PICVA)*—Flow redirection from diseased coronary artery into adjacent coronary vein, causing arterialisation of the vein and retroperfusion into ischaemic myocardium
- *Percutaneous in situ coronary artery bypass (PICAB)*—Flow redirection from diseased artery into adjacent coronary vein and then rerouted back into the artery after the lesion
- *Heart transplantation*—May be considered when all alternative treatments have failed

Further reading
- Yusuf S, Zucker D, Peduzzi P, Fisher LD, Takaro T, Kennedy JW, et al. Effect of coronary artery bypass graft surgery on survival; overview of 10-year results from randomised trials by the Coronary Artery Bypass Graft Surgery Trialists Collaboration. *Lancet* 1994; 344: 563-70
- Pocock SJ, Henderson RA, Rickards AF, Hampton JR, King SB 3rd, Hamm CW, et al. Meta-analysis of randomised trials comparing coronary angioplasty with bypass surgery. *Lancet* 1995;345:1184-9
- Raco DL, Yusuf S. Overview of randomised trials of percutaneous coronary intervention: comparison with medical and surgical therapy for chronic coronary artery disease. In: Grech ED, Ramsdale DR, eds. *Practical interventional cardiology*. 2nd ed. London: Martin Dunitz, 2002:263-77
- Serruys PW, Unger F, Sousa JE, Jatene A, Bonnier HJ, Schonberger JP, et al for the Arterial Revascularisation Therapies Study (ARTS) Group. Comparison of coronary-artery bypass surgery and stenting for multivessel disease. *N Engl J Med* 2001;344:1117-24
- Kim MC, Kini A, Sharma SK. Refractory angina pectoris. Mechanisms and therapeutic options. *J Am Coll Cardiol* 2002;39: 923-34
- Morice M-C, Serruys PW, Sousa JE, Fajadet J, Ban Hayashi E, Perin M, et al. A randomized comparison of a sirolimus-eluting stent with a standard stent for coronary revascularization. *N Engl J Med* 2002;346:1773-80
- Scottish Intercollegiate Guidelines Network. *Coronary revascularisation in the management of stable angina pectoris.* Edinburgh: SIGN, 1998 (SIGN Publication No 32)

5 Acute coronary syndrome: unstable angina and non-ST segment elevation myocardial infarction

Ever D Grech, David R Ramsdale

The term acute coronary syndrome refers to a range of acute myocardial ischaemic states. It encompasses unstable angina, non-ST segment elevation myocardial infarction (ST segment elevation generally absent), and ST segment elevation infarction (persistent ST segment elevation usually present). This article will focus on the role of percutaneous coronary intervention in the management of unstable angina and non-ST segment elevation myocardial infarction; the next article will address the role of percutaneous intervention in ST segment elevation infarction.

Although there is no universally accepted definition of unstable angina, it has been described as a clinical syndrome between stable angina and acute myocardial infarction. This broad definition encompasses many patients presenting with varying histories and reflects the complex pathophysiological mechanisms operating at different times and with different outcomes. Three main presentations have been described—angina at rest, new onset angina, and increasing angina.

Pathogenesis

The process central to the initiation of an acute coronary syndrome is disruption of an atheromatous plaque. Fissuring or rupture of these plaques—and consequent exposure of core constituents such as lipid, smooth muscle, and foam cells—leads to the local generation of thrombin and deposition of fibrin. This in turn promotes platelet aggregation and adhesion and the formation of intracoronary thrombus.

Unstable angina and non-ST segment elevation myocardial infarction are generally associated with white, platelet-rich, and only partially occlusive thrombus. Microthrombi can detach and embolise downstream, causing myocardial ischaemia and infarction. In contrast, ST segment elevation (or Q wave) myocardial infarction has red, fibrin-rich, and more stable occlusive thrombus.

Epidemiology

Unstable angina and non-ST segment elevation myocardial infarction account for about 2.5 million hospital admissions worldwide and are a major cause of mortality and morbidity in Western countries. The prognosis is substantially worse than for chronic stable angina. In-hospital death and re-infarction affect 5-10%. Despite optimal treatment with anti-ischaemic and antithrombotic drugs, death and recurrent myocardial infarction occur in another 5-10% of patients in the month after an acute episode. Several studies indicate that these patients may have a higher long term risk of death and myocardial infarction than do patients with ST segment elevation.

Diagnosis

Unstable angina and non-ST segment elevation myocardial infarction are closely related conditions with clinical presentations that may be indistinguishable. Their distinction depends on whether the ischaemia is severe enough to cause myocardial damage and the release of detectable quantities of

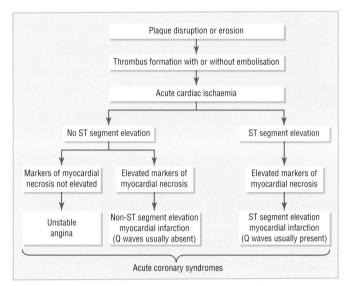

Spectrum of acute coronary syndromes according to electrocardiographic and biochemical markers of myocardial necrosis (troponin T, troponin I, and creatine kinase MB), in patients presenting with acute cardiac chest pain

---

Three main presentations of unstable angina

- *Angina at rest*—Also prolonged, usually >20 minutes
- *Angina of new onset*—At least CCS class III in severity
- *Angina increasing*—Previously diagnosed angina that has become more frequent, longer in duration, or lower in threshold (change in severity by ≥1 CCS class to at least CCS class III)

CCS=Canadian Cardiovascular Society

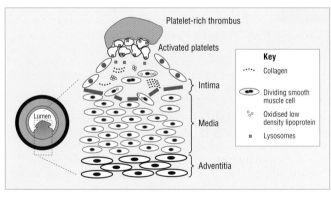

Diagram of an unstable plaque with superimposed luminal thrombus

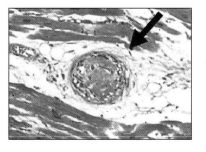

Distal embolisation of a platelet-rich thrombus causing occlusion of intramyocardial arteriole (arrow). Such an event may result in micro-infarction and elevation of markers of myocardial necrosis

markers of myocyte necrosis. Cardiac troponin I and T are the preferred markers as they are more specific and reliable than creatine kinase or its isoenzyme creatine kinase MB.

An electrocardiogram may be normal or show minor non-specific changes, ST segment depression, T wave inversion, bundle branch block, or transient ST segment elevation that resolves spontaneously or after nitrate is given. Physical examination may exclude important differential diagnoses such as pleuritis, pericarditis, or pneumothorax, as well as revealing evidence of ventricular failure and haemodynamic instability.

Management

Management has evolved considerably over the past decade. As platelet aggregation and thrombus formation play a key role in acute coronary syndrome, recent advances in treatment (such as the glycoprotein IIb/IIIa inhibitors, low molecular weight heparin, and clopidogrel) and the safer and more widespread use of percutaneous coronary intervention have raised questions about optimal management.

As patients with unstable angina or non-ST segment elevation myocardial infarction represent a heterogeneous group with a wide spectrum of clinical outcomes, tailoring treatment to match risk not only ensures that patients who will benefit the most receive appropriate treatment, but also avoids potentially hazardous treatment in those with a good prognosis. Therefore, an accurate diagnosis and estimation of the risk of adverse outcome are prerequisites to selecting the most appropriate treatment. This should begin in the emergency department and continue throughout the hospital admission. Ideally, all patients should be assessed by a cardiologist on the day of presentation.

Medical treatment

Medical treatment includes bed rest, oxygen, opiate analgesics to relieve pain, and anti-ischaemic and antithrombotic drugs. These should be started at once on admission and continued in those with probable or confirmed unstable angina or non-ST segment elevation myocardial infarction. Anti-ischaemic drugs include intravenous, oral, or buccal nitroglycerin, β blockers, and calcium antagonists. Antithrombotic drugs include aspirin, clopidogrel, intravenous unfractionated heparin or low molecular weight heparin, and glycoprotein IIb/IIIa inhibitors.

Conservative versus early invasive strategy

"Conservative" treatment involves intensive medical management, followed by risk stratification by non-invasive means (usually by stress testing) to identify patients who may need coronary angiography. This approach is based on the results of two randomised trials (TIMI IIIB and VANQWISH), which showed no improvement in outcome when an "early invasive" strategy was used routinely, compared with a selective approach.

These findings generated much controversy and have been superseded by more recent randomised trials (FRISC II, TACTICS-TIMI 18, and RITA 3), which have taken advantage of the benefits of glycoprotein IIb/IIIa inhibitors and stents. All three studies showed that an early invasive strategy (percutaneous coronary intervention or coronary artery bypass surgery) produced a better outcome than non-invasive management. TACTICS-TIMI 18 also showed that the benefit of early invasive treatment was greatest in higher risk patients with raised plasma concentrations of troponin T, whereas the outcomes for lower risk patients were similar with early invasive and non-invasive management.

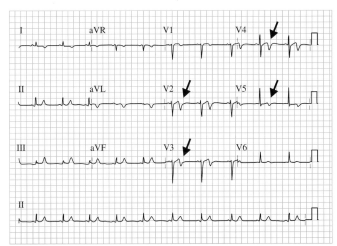

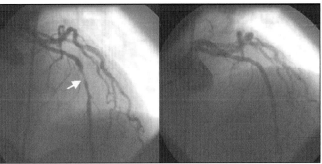

Electrocardiogram of a 48 year old woman with unstable angina (top). Note the acute ischaemic changes in leads V1 to V5 (arrows). Coronary angiography revealed a severe mid-left anterior descending coronary artery stenosis (arrow, bottom left), which was successfully stented (bottom right)

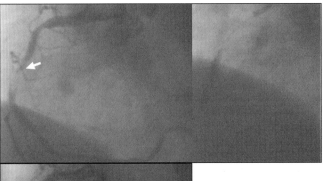

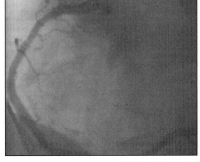

Right coronary artery angiogram in patient with non-ST segment elevation myocardial infarction (top left), showing hazy appearance of intraluminal thrombus overlying a severe stenosis (arrow). Abciximab was given before direct stenting (top right), with good angiographic outcome (bottom)

Names of trials

- TIMI IIIB—Thrombolysis in myocardial infarction IIIB
- VANQWISH—Veterans affairs non-Q-wave infarction strategies in hospital
- GUSTO IV ACS—Global use of strategies to open occluded arteries-IV in acute coronary syndromes
- RITA 3—Randomised intervention treatment of angina
- FRISC II—Fast revascularisation during instability in coronary artery disease
- TACTICS-TIMI 18—Treat angina with Aggrastat and determine cost of therapy with an invasive or conservative strategy-thrombolysis in myocardial infarction

Identifying higher risk patients

Identifying patients at higher risk of death, myocardial infarction, and recurrent ischaemia allows aggressive antithrombotic treatment and early coronary angiography to be targeted to those who will benefit. The initial diagnosis is made on the basis of a patient's history, electrocardiography, and the presence of elevated plasma concentrations of biochemical markers. The same information is used to assess the risk of an adverse outcome. It should be emphasised that risk assessment is a continuous process.

The TIMI risk score

Attempts have been made to formulate clinical factors into a user friendly model. Notably, Antman and colleagues identified seven independent prognostic risk factors for early death and myocardial infarction. Assigning a value of 1 for each risk factor present provides a simple scoring system for estimating risk, the TIMI risk score. It has the advantage of being easy to calculate and has broad applicability in the early assessment of patients.

Applying this score to the results in the TACTICS-TIMI 18 study indicated that patients with a TIMI risk score of ≥3 benefited significantly from an early invasive strategy, whereas those with a score of ≤2 did not. Therefore, those with an initial TIMI score of ≥3 should be considered for early angiography (ideally within 24 hours), with a view to revascularisation by percutaneous intervention or bypass surgery. In addition, any patient with an elevated plasma concentration of troponin marker, ST segment changes, or haemodynamic instability should also undergo early angiography.

Conclusion

The diagnosis of unstable angina or non-ST segment elevation myocardial infarction demands urgent hospital admission and coronary monitoring. A clinical history and examination, 12 lead electrocardiography, and measurement of troponin concentration are the essential diagnostic tools. Bed rest, aspirin, clopidogrel, heparin, antianginal drugs, and opiate analgesics are the mainstay of initial treatment.

Early risk stratification will help identify high risk patients, who may require early treatment with glycoprotein IIb/IIIa inhibitors, angiography, and coronary revascularisation. Those deemed suitable for percutaneous intervention should receive a glycoprotein IIb/IIIa inhibitor and stenting as appropriate. There seems to be little merit in prolonged stabilisation of patients before percutaneous intervention, and an early invasive strategy is generally preferable to a conservative one except for patients at low risk of further cardiac events. This approach will shorten hospital stays, improve acute and long term outcomes, and reduce the need for subsequent intervention.

In the longer term, aggressive modification of risk factors is warranted. Smoking should be strongly discouraged, and statins should be used to lower blood lipid levels. Long term treatment with aspirin, clopidogrel (especially after stenting), β blockers, angiotensin converting enzyme inhibitors, and antihypertensive drugs should also be considered. Anti-ischaemic drugs may be stopped when ischaemia provocation tests are negative.

The picture of a microthrombus occluding an intramyocardial arteriole was provided by K MacDonald, consultant histopathologist, St Boniface Hospital, Winnipeg.

Competing interests: None declared.

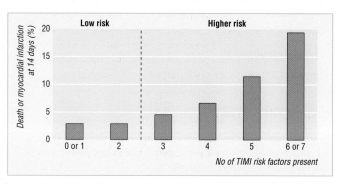

Rates of death from all causes and non-fatal myocardial infarction at 14 days, by TIMI risk score. Note sharp rate increase when score ≥3

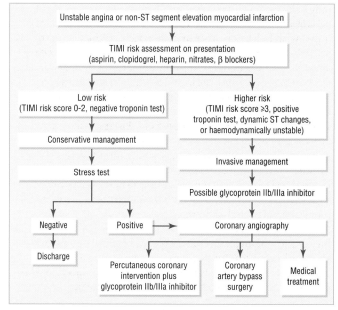

Simplified management pathway for patients with unstable angina or non-ST segment elevation myocardial infarction

Further reading

- Braunwald E, Antman EM, Beasley JW, Califf RM, Cheitlin MD, Hochman JS, et al. ACC/AHA 2002 guideline update for the management of patients with unstable angina and non-ST-segment elevation myocardial infarction: a report of the American College of Cardiology/American Heart Association task force on practice guidelines. *J Am Coll Cardiol* 2002;40:1366-74
- Bertrand ME, Simoons ML, Fox KA, Wallentin LC, Hamm CW, McFadden E, et al. Management of acute coronary syndromes: acute coronary syndromes without persistent ST segment elevation. Recommendations of the Task Force of the European Society of Cardiology. *Eur Heart J* 2000;21:1406-32
- Antman EM, Cohen M, Bernink PJ, McCabe CH, Horacek T, Papuchis G, et al. The TIMI risk score for unstable angina/non-ST elevation MI: a method for prognostication and therapeutic decision making. *JAMA* 2000;284:835-42
- Ramsdale DR, Grech ED. Percutaneous coronary intervention unstable angina and non-Q-wave myocardial infarction. In: Grech ED, Ramsdale DR, eds. *Practical interventional cardiology*. 2nd ed. London: Martin Dunitz, 2002:165-87

6 Acute coronary syndrome: ST segment elevation myocardial infarction

Ever D Grech, David R Ramsdale

Acute ST segment elevation myocardial infarction usually occurs when thrombus forms on a ruptured atheromatous plaque and occludes an epicardial coronary artery. Patient survival depends on several factors, the most important being restoration of brisk antegrade coronary flow, the time taken to achieve this, and the sustained patency of the affected artery.

Recanalisation

There are two main methods of re-opening an occluded artery: administering a thrombolytic agent or primary percutaneous transluminal coronary angioplasty.

Although thrombolysis is the commonest form of treatment for acute myocardial infarction, it has important limitations: a rate of recanalisation (restoring normal flow) in 90 minutes of only 55% with streptokinase or 60% with accelerated alteplase; a 5-15% risk of early or late reocclusion leading to acute myocardial infarction, worsening ventricular function, or death; a 1-2% risk of intracranial haemorrhage, with 40% mortality; and 15-20% of patients with a contraindication to thrombolysis.

Primary angioplasty (also called direct angioplasty) mechanically disrupts the occlusive thrombus and compresses the underlying stenosis, rapidly restoring blood flow. It offers a superior alternative to thrombolysis in the immediate treatment of ST segment elevation myocardial infarction. This differs from sequential angioplasty, when angioplasty is performed after thrombolysis. After early trials of thrombolytic drugs, there was much interest in "adjunctive" angioplasty (angioplasty used as a supplement to successful thrombolysis) as this was expected to reduce recurrent ischaemia and re-infarction. Later studies, however, not only failed to show any advantage, but found higher rates of major haemorrhage and emergency bypass surgery. In contrast, "rescue" (also known as "salvage") angioplasty, which is performed if thrombolysis fails to restore patency after one to two hours, may confer benefit.

Pros and cons of primary angioplasty

Advantages
Large randomised studies have shown that thrombolysis significantly reduces mortality compared with placebo, and this effect is maintained long term. Primary angioplasty confers

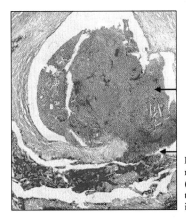

Histological appearance of a ruptured atheromatous plaque (bottom arrow) and occlusive thrombus (top arrow) resulting in acute myocardial infarction

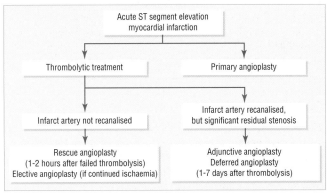

Methods of recanalisation for acute myocardial infarction

Comparison of methods of recanalisation

	Thrombolysis	Rescue angioplasty	Primary angioplasty
Time from admission to recanalisation	1-3 hours after start of thrombolysis	Time to start of thrombolysis plus 2 hours	20-60 minutes
Recanalisation with brisk antegrade flow	55-60%	85%	95%
Systemic fibrinolysis	+++	+++	−
Staff and catheter laboratory "burden"	−	+	+++
Cost of procedure	+	+++	+++

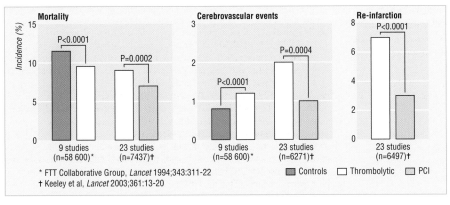

Effects of treatment with placebo, thrombolytic drugs, or primary percutaneous coronary intervention (PCI) on mortality, incidence of cerebrovascular events, and incidence of non-fatal re-infarction after acute myocardial infarction in randomised studies. Of the 1% incidence of cerebrovascular events in patients undergoing primary percutaneous intervention, only 0.05% were haemorrhagic. In contrast patients receiving thrombolytic drugs had a 1% incidence of haemorrhagic cerebrovascular events (P<0.0001) and an overall 2% incidence of cerebrovascular events (P=0.0004)

19

extra benefits in terms of substantial reductions in rates of death, cerebrovascular events, and re-infarction.

The information provided by immediate coronary angiography is valuable in determining subsequent management. Patients with severe three vessel disease, severe left main coronary artery stenosis, or occluded vessels unsuitable for angioplasty can be referred for bypass surgery. Conversely, patients whose arteries are found to have spontaneously recanalised or who have an insignificant infarct related artery may be selected for medical treatment, and thus avoid unnecessary thrombolytic treatment.

Disadvantages

The morbidity and mortality associated with primary angioplasty is operator dependent, varying with the skill and experience of the interventionist, and it should be considered only for patients presenting early (< 12 hours after acute myocardial infarction).

Procedural complications are more common than with elective angioplasty for chronic angina, and, even though it is usual to deal only with the occluded vessel, procedures may be prolonged. Ventricular arrhythmias are not unusual on recanalisation, but these generally occur while the patient is still in the catheterisation laboratory and can be promptly treated by intravenous drugs or electrical cardioversion. Right coronary artery procedures are often associated with sinus arrest, atrioventricular block, idioventricular rhythm, and severe hypotension. Up to 5% of patients initially referred for primary angioplasty require urgent coronary artery bypass surgery, so surgical backup is essential if risks are to be minimised.

There are logistical hurdles in delivering a full 24 hour service. Primary angioplasty can be performed only when adequate facilities and experienced staff are available. The time from admission to recanalisation should be less than 60 minutes, which may not be possible if staff are on call from home. However, recent evidence suggests that, even with longer delays, primary angioplasty may still be superior to thrombolysis.

A catheterisation laboratory requires large initial capital expenditure and has substantial running costs. However, in an existing, fully supported laboratory operating at high volume, primary angioplasty is at least as cost effective as thrombolysis.

Primary angioplasty and coronary stents

Although early randomised studies of primary angioplasty showed its clinical effectiveness, outcomes were marred by high rates of recurrent ischaemia (10-15% of patients) and early reinfarction of the affected artery (up to 5%). Consequently, haemodynamic and arrhythmic complications arose, with the need for repeat catheterisation and revascularisation, prolonged hospital stay, and increased costs. Furthermore, restenosis rates in the first six months remained disappointingly high (25-45%), and a fifth of patients required revascularisation.

Although stenting the lesion seemed an attractive answer, it was initially thought that deploying a stent in the presence of thrombus over a ruptured plaque would provoke further thrombosis. However, improvements in stent deployment and advances in adjunctive pharmacotherapy have led to greater technical success. Recent studies comparing primary stenting with balloon angioplasty alone have shown that stented patients have significantly less recurrent ischaemia, reinfarction, and subsequent need for further angioplasty. Economic analysis has shown that, as expected, the initial costs were higher but were offset by lower follow up costs after a year.

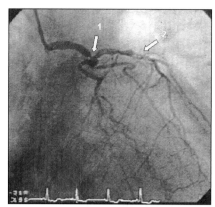

Severe distal left main stem stenosis (arrow 1) and partially occluded mid-left anterior descending artery due to thrombus (arrow 2). In view of the severity of the lesion salvage angioplasty was contraindicated. An intra-aortic balloon pump was used to augment blood pressure and coronary flow before successful bypass surgery

---

Pros and cons of primary angioplasty* compared with thrombolysis

Advantages
- High patency rates (> 90%) with brisk, antegrade flow
- Lower mortality
- Better residual left ventricular function
- More rapid electrocardiographic normalisation
- Less recurrent ischaemia (angina, reinfarction, exercise induced ischaemia)
- No systemic fibrinolysis, therefore bleeding problems avoided
- Improved risk stratification by angiography with identification of patients suitable for coronary artery bypass surgery

Disadvantages
- Higher procedural cost than streptokinase or alteplase (although long term costs lower)
- Can be performed only when cardiac catheterisation facilities and experienced staff available
- Recanalisation more rapid than thrombolysis only if 24 hour on-call team available
- Risks and complications of cardiac catheterisation and percutaneous intervention
- Reperfusion arrhythmias probably more common because of more rapid recanalisation

*With or without stenting

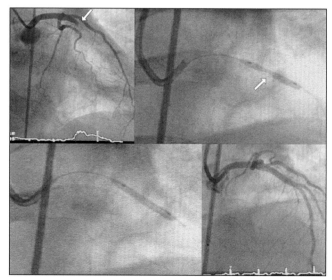

Anterior myocardial infarction of 4 hours' duration and severe hypotension, caused by a totally occluded proximal left anterior descending artery (arrow, top left). After treatment with abciximab, a stent was positioned. Initial inflation showed "waisting" of the balloon (top right), due to fibrous lesion resistance, which resolved on higher inflation (bottom left). Successful recanalisation resulted in brisk flow (bottom right), and the 15 minute procedure completely resolved the patient's chest pain

However, one study (Stent-PAMI) showed that stenting was associated with a small (but significant) decrease in normal coronary flow and a trend towards increased six and 12 month mortality. This led some to examine the use of adjunctive glycoprotein IIb/IIIa inhibitors as a solution.

Stenting and glycoprotein IIb/IIIa inhibitors

The first study (CADILLAC) to examine the potential benefits of glycoprotein IIb/IIIa inhibitors combined with stenting showed that abciximab significantly reduced early recurrent ischaemia and reocclusion due to thrombus formation. There was no additional effect on restenosis or late outcomes compared with stenting alone. The slightly reduced rate of normal coronary flow that had been seen in other studies was again confirmed, but did not translate into a significant effect on mortality.

Another study (ADMIRAL) examined the potential benefit of abciximab when given before (rather than during) primary stenting. Both at 30 days' and six months' follow up, abciximab significantly reduced the composite rate of reinfarction, the need for further revascularisation, and mortality. In addition, abciximab significantly improved coronary flow rates immediately after stenting, which persisted up to six months with a significant improvement in residual left ventricular function.

Future of primary angioplasty

Primary stenting is not only safe but, by reducing recurrent ischaemic events, also confers advantages over balloon angioplasty alone. Abciximab treatment seems to further improve flow characteristics, prevents distal thrombo-embolisation, and reduces the need for repeat angioplasty. A strategy of primary stenting in association with abciximab seems to be the current gold standard of care for patients with acute myocardial infarction. Future studies will examine the potential benefit of other glycoprotein IIb/IIIa inhibitors. The question of whether on-site surgical cover is still essential for infarct intervention continues to be debated.

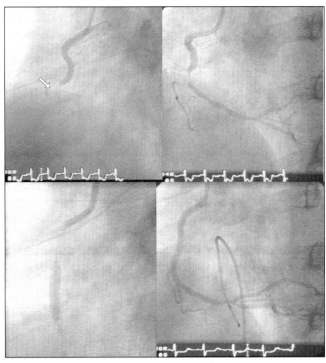

Inferior myocardial infarction of 2.5 hours' duration caused by a totally occluded middle right coronary artery (arrow, top left). A guide wire passed through the fresh thrombus produced slow distal filling (top right). Deployment of a stent (bottom left) resulted in brisk antegrade flow, a good angiographic result, and relief of chest pain (bottom right). A temporary pacemaker electrode was used to counter a reperfusion junctional bradycardia. Note resolution in ST segments compared with top angiograms

Names of trials

- CADILLAC—Controlled abciximab and device investigation to lower late angioplasty complications
- ADMIRAL—Abciximab before direct angioplasty and stenting in myocardial infarction regarding acute and long-term follow-up
- Stent-PAMI—Stent primary angioplasty in myocardial infarction

Further reading

- Fibrinolytic Therapy Trialists' (FTT) Collaborative Group. Indications for fibrinolytic therapy in suspected acute myocardial infarction: collaborative overview of early mortality and major morbidity results from all randomised trials of more than 1000 patients. *Lancet* 1994;343:311-22
- Keeley EC, Boura JA, Grines CL. Primary angioplasty versus intravenous thrombolytic therapy for acute myocardial infarction: a quantitative review of 23 randomised trials. *Lancet* 2003;361:13-20
- De Boer MJ, Zijlstra F. Coronary angioplasty in acute myocardial infarction. In: Grech ED, Ramsdale DR, eds. *Practical interventional cardiology*. 2nd ed. London: Martin Dunitz, 2002:189-206
- Lieu TA, Gurley RJ, Lundstrom RJ, Ray GT, Fireman BH, Weinstein MC, et al. Projected cost-effectiveness of primary angioplasty for acute myocardial infarction. *J Am Coll Cardiol* 1997;30:1741-50
- Grines CL, Cox DA, Stone GW, Garcia E, Mattos LA, Giambartolomei A, et al, for the Stent Primary Angioplasty in Myocardial Infarction Study Group. Coronary angioplasty with or without stent implantation for acute myocardial infarction. *N Engl J Med* 1999;341: 1949-56
- Montalescot G, Barragan P, Wittenberg O, Ecollan P, Elhadad S, Villain P, et al. Platelet glycoprotein IIb/IIIa inhibition with coronary stenting for acute myocardial infarction. *N Engl J Med* 2001;344:1895-903
- Stone GW, Grines CL, Cox DA, Garcia E, Tcheng JE, Griffin JJ, et al. Comparison of angioplasty with stenting, with or without abciximab, in acute myocardial infarction. *N Engl J Med* 2002;346:957-66

7 Percutaneous coronary intervention: cardiogenic shock

John Ducas, Ever D Grech

Cardiogenic shock is the commonest cause of death after acute myocardial infarction. It occurs in 7% of patients with ST segment elevation myocardial infarction and 3% with non-ST segment elevation myocardial infarction.

Cardiogenic shock is a progressive state of hypotension (systolic blood pressure <90 mm Hg) lasting at least 30 minutes, despite adequate preload and heart rate, which leads to systemic hypoperfusion. It is usually caused by left ventricular systolic dysfunction. A patient requiring drug or mechanical support to maintain a systolic blood pressure over 90 mm Hg can also be considered as manifesting cardiogenic shock. As cardiac output and blood pressure fall, there is an increase in sympathetic tone, with subsequent cardiac and systemic effects—such as altered mental state, cold extremities, peripheral cyanosis, and urine output <30 ml/hour.

Effects of cardiogenic shock

Cardiac effects
In an attempt to maintain cardiac output, the remaining non-ischaemic myocardium becomes hypercontractile, and its oxygen consumption increases. The effectiveness of this response depends on the extent of current and previous left ventricular damage, the severity of coexisting coronary artery disease, and the presence of other cardiac pathology such as valve disease.

Three possible outcomes may occur:
● Compensation—which restores normal blood pressure and myocardial perfusion pressure
● Partial compensation—which results in a pre-shock state with mildly depressed cardiac output and blood pressure, as well as an elevated heart rate and left ventricular filling pressure
● Shock—which develops rapidly and leads to profound hypotension and worsening global myocardial ischaemia. Without immediate reperfusion, patients in this group have little potential for myocardial salvage or survival.

Systemic effects
The falling blood pressure increases catecholamine levels, leading to systemic arterial and venous constriction. In time, activation of the renin-aldosterone-angiotensin axis causes further vasoconstriction, with subsequent sodium and water retention. These responses have the effect of increasing left ventricular filling pressure and volume. Although this partly compensates for the decline in left ventricular function, a high left ventricular filling pressure leads to pulmonary oedema, which impairs gas exchange. The ensuing respiratory acidosis exacerbates cardiac ischaemia, left ventricular dysfunction, and intravascular thrombosis.

Time course of cardiogenic shock
The onset of cardiogenic shock is variable. In the GUSTO-I study, of patients with acute myocardial infarction, 7% developed cardiogenic shock—11% on admission and 89% in the subsequent two weeks. Almost all of those who developed cardiogenic shock did so by 48 hours after the onset of symptoms, and their overall 30 day mortality was 57%, compared with an overall study group mortality of just 7%.

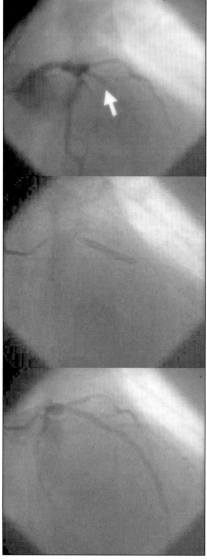

A 65 year old man with a 3-4 hour history of acute anterior myocardial infarction had cardiogenic shock and acute pulmonary oedema, requiring mechanical ventilation and inotropic support. He underwent emergency angiography (top), which showed a totally occluded proximal left anterior descending artery (arrow). A soft tipped guidewire was passed across the occlusive thrombotic lesion, which was successfully stented (middle). Restoration of brisk antegrade flow down this artery (bottom) followed by insertion of an intra-aortic balloon pump markedly improved blood pressure and organ perfusion. The next day he was extubated and weaned off all inotropic drugs, and the intra-aortic balloon pump was removed

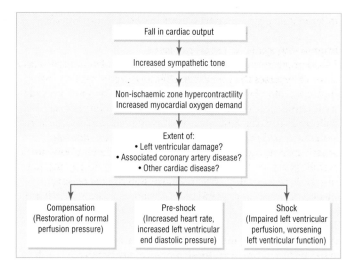

Cardiac compensatory response to falling cardiac output after acute myocardial infarction.

22

Differential diagnosis

Hypotension can complicate acute myocardial infarction in other settings.

Right coronary artery occlusion

An occluded right coronary artery (which usually supplies a smaller proportion of the left ventricular muscle than the left coronary artery) may lead to hypotension in various ways: cardiac output can fall due to vagally mediated reflex venodilatation and bradycardia, and right ventricular dilation may displace the intraventricular septum towards the left ventricular cavity, preventing proper filling.

In addition, the right coronary artery occasionally supplies a sizeable portion of left ventricular myocardium. In this case right ventricular myocardial infarction produces a unique set of physical findings, haemodynamic characteristics, and ST segment elevation in lead V_4R. When this occurs aggressive treatment is indicated as the mortality exceeds 30%.

Ventricular septal defect, mitral regurgitation, or myocardial rupture

In 10% of patients with cardiogenic shock, hypotension arises from a ventricular septal defect induced by myocardial infarction or severe mitral regurgitation after papillary muscle rupture. Such a condition should be suspected if a patient develops a new systolic murmur, and is readily confirmed by echocardiography—which should be urgently requested. Such patients have high mortality, and urgent referral for surgery may be needed. Even with surgery, the survival rate can be low.

Myocardial rupture of the free wall may cause low cardiac output as a result of cardiac compression due to tamponade. It is more difficult to diagnose clinically (raised venous pressure, pulsus paradoxus), but the presence of haemopericardium can be readily confirmed by echocardiography. Pericardial aspiration often leads to rapid increase in cardiac output, and surgery may be necessary.

Management

The left ventricular filling volume should be optimised, and in the absence of pulmonary congestion a saline fluid challenge of at least 250 ml should be administered over 10 minutes. Adequate oxygenation is crucial, and intubation or ventilation should be used early if gas exchange abnormalities are present. Ongoing hypotension induces respiratory muscle failure, and this is prevented with mechanical ventilation. Antithrombotic treatment (aspirin and intravenous heparin) is appropriate.

Supporting systemic blood pressure

Blood pressure support maintains perfusion of vital organs and slows or reverses the metabolic effects of organ hypoperfusion. Inotropes stimulate myocardial function and increase vascular tone, allowing perfusion pressures to increase. Intra-aortic balloon pump counterpulsation often has a dramatic effect on systemic blood pressure. Inflation occurs in early diastole, greatly increasing aortic diastolic pressure to levels above aortic systolic pressure. In addition, balloon deflation during the start of systole reduces the aortic pressure, thereby decreasing myocardial oxygen demand and forward resistance (afterload).

Reperfusion

Although inotropic drugs and mechanical support increase systemic blood pressure, these measures are temporary and have no effect on long term survival unless they are combined with coronary artery recanalisation and myocardial reperfusion.

Hallmarks of right ventricular infarction

- Rising jugular venous pressure, Kassmaul sign, pulsus paradoxus
- Low output with little pulmonary congestion
- Right atrial pressure >10 mm Hg and >80% of pulmonary capillary wedge pressure
- Right atrial prominent Y descent
- Right ventricle shows dip and plateau pattern of pressure
- Profound hypoxia with right to left shunt through a patent foramen ovale
- ST segment elevation in lead V_4R

Main indications and contraindications for intra-aortic balloon pump counterpulsation

Indications

- Cardiogenic shock
- Unstable and refractory angina
- Cardiac support for high risk percutaneous intervention
- Hypoperfusion after coronary artery bypass graft surgery
- Septic shock
- Enhancement of coronary flow after succesful recanalisation by percutaneous intervention
- Ventricular septal defect and papillary muscle rupture after myocardial infarction
- Intractable ischaemic ventricular tachycardia

Contraindications

- Severe aortic regurgitation
- Abdominal or aortic aneurysm
- Severe aorto-iliac disease or peripheral vascular disease

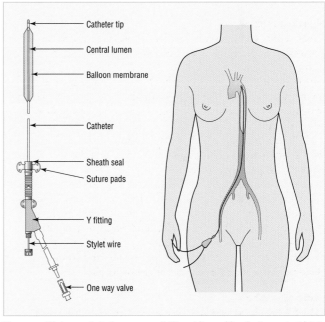

Diagram of intra-aortic balloon pump (left) and its position in the aorta (right)

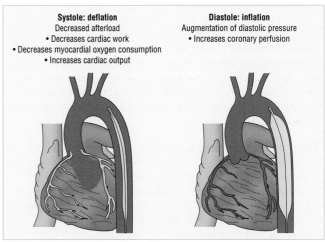

Effects of intra-aortic balloon pump during systole and diastole

Thrombolysis is currently the commonest form of treatment for myocardial infarction. However, successful fibrinolysis probably depends on drug delivery to the clot, and as blood pressure falls, so reperfusion becomes less likely. One study (GISSI) showed that, in patients with cardiogenic shock, streptokinase conferred no benefit compared with placebo.

The GUSTO-I investigators examined data on 2200 patients who either presented with cardiogenic shock or who developed it after enrolment and survived for at least an hour after its onset. Thirty day mortality was considerably less in those undergoing early angiography (38%) than in patients with late or no angiography (62%). Further analysis suggested that early angiography was independently associated with a 43% reduction in 30 day mortality.

In the SHOCK trial, patients with cardiogenic shock were treated aggressively with inotropic drugs, intra-aortic balloon pump counterpulsation, and thrombolytic drugs. Patients were also randomised to either coronary angiography plus percutaneous intervention or bypass surgery within six hours, or medical stabilisation (with revascularisation only permitted after 54 hours). Although the 30 day primary end point did not achieve statistical significance, the death rates progressively diverged, and by 12 months the early revascularisation group showed a significant mortality benefit (55%) compared with the medical stabilisation group (70%). The greatest benefit was seen in those aged < 75 years and those treated early (< 6 hours). Given an absolute risk reduction of 15% at 12 months, one life would be saved for only seven patients treated by aggressive, early revascularisation.

Support and reperfusion: impact on survival

Over the past 10 years, specific measures to improve blood pressure and restore arterial perfusion have been instituted. Mortality data collected since the 1970s show a significant fall in mortality in the 1990s corresponding with increased use of combinations of thrombolytic drugs, the intra-aortic balloon pump, and coronary angiography with revascularisation by either percutaneous intervention or bypass surgery. Before these measures, death rates of 80% were consistently observed.

Cardiogenic shock is the commonest cause of death in acute myocardial infarction. Although thrombolysis can be attempted with inotropic support or augmentation of blood pressure with the intra-aortic balloon pump, the greatest mortality benefit is seen after urgent coronary angiography and revascularisation. Cardiogenic shock is a catheter laboratory emergency.

The diagram of patient mortality after myocardial infarction is adapted with permission from Goldberg RJ et al, *N Engl J Med* 1999;340:1162-8.

Competing interests: None declared.

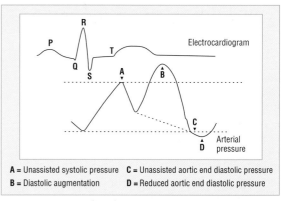

A = Unassisted systolic pressure   C = Unassisted aortic end diastolic pressure
B = Diastolic augmentation   D = Reduced aortic end diastolic pressure

Diagram of electrocardiogram and aortic pressure wave showing timing of intra-aortic balloon pump and its effects of diastolic augmentation (D) and reduced aortic end diastolic pressure

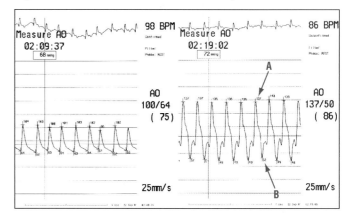

Aortic pressure wave recording before (left) and during (right) intra-aortic balloon pump counterpulsation in a patient with cardiogenic shock after myocardial infarction. Note marked augmentation in diastolic pressure (arrow A) and reduction in end diastolic pressures (arrow B). (AO=aortic pressure)

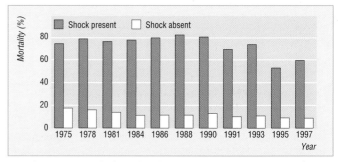

Mortality after myocardial infarction with or without cardiogenic shock (1975 to 1997). Mortality of patients in shock fell from roughly 80% to 60% in the 1990s

Names of trials

- GISSI—Gruppo Italiano per lo studio della sopravvivenza nell'infarto miocardico
- GUSTO—global utilization of streptokinase and tissue plasminogen activator for occluded coronary arteries
- SHOCK—should we emergently revascularize occluded coronaries for cardiogenic shock

Further reading

- Hochman JS, Sleeper LA, Webb JG, Sanborn TA, White HD, Talley JD, et al. Early revascularization in acute myocardial infarction complicated by cardiogenic shock. *N Engl J Med* 1999;341:625-34
- Berger PB, Holmes DR Jr, Stebbins AL, Bates ER, Califf RM, Topol EJ. Impact of an aggressive invasive catheterization and revascularization strategy on mortality in patients with cardiogenic shock in the global utilization of streptokinase and tissue plasminogen activator for occluded coronary arteries (GUSTO-I) trial. *Circulation* 1997;96:122-7

- Golberg RJ, Samad NA, Yarzebski J, Gurwitz J, Bigelow C, Gore JM. Temporal trends in cardiogenic shock complicating acute myocardial infarction. *N Engl J Med* 1999;340:1162-8
- Hasdai D, Topol EJ, Califf RM, Berger PB, Holmes DR. Cardiogenic shock complicating acute coronary syndromes. *Lancet* 2000;356:749-56
- White HD. Cardiogenic shock: a more aggressive approach is now warranted. *Eur Heart J* 2000;21:1897-901

8 Interventional pharmacotherapy

Roger Philipp, Ever D Grech

The dramatic increase in the use of percutaneous coronary intervention has been possible because of advances in adjunctive pharmacotherapy, which have greatly improved safety. Percutaneous intervention inevitably causes vessel trauma, with disruption of the endothelium and atheromatous plaque. This activates prothrombotic factors, leading to localised thrombosis; this may impair blood flow, precipitate vessel occlusion, or cause distal embolisation. Coronary stents exacerbate this problem as they are thrombogenic. For these reasons, drug inhibition of thrombus formation during percutaneous coronary intervention is mandatory, although this must be balanced against the risk of bleeding, both systemic and at the access site.

Coronary artery thrombosis

Platelets are central to thrombus formation. Vessel trauma during percutaneous intervention exposes subendothelial collagen and von Willebrand factor, which activate platelet surface receptors and induce the initial steps of platelet activation. Further platelet activation ultimately results in activation of platelet glycoprotein IIb/IIIa receptor—the final common pathway for platelet aggregation.

Vascular injury and membrane damage also trigger coagulation by exposure of tissue factors. The resulting thrombin formation further activates platelets and converts fibrinogen to fibrin. The final event is the binding of fibrinogen to activated glycoprotein IIb/IIIa receptors to form a platelet aggregate.

Understanding of these mechanisms has led to the development of potent anticoagulants and antiplatelet inhibitors that can be used for percutaneous coronary intervention. Since the early days of percutaneous transluminal coronary angioplasty, heparin and aspirin have remained a fundamental part of percutaneous coronary intervention treatment. Following the introduction of stents, ticlopidine and more recently clopidogrel have allowed a very low rate of stent thrombosis. More recently, glycoprotein IIb/IIIa receptor antagonists have reduced procedural complications still further and improved the protection of the distal microcirculation, especially in thrombus-containing lesions prevalent in acute coronary syndromes.

Antithrombotic therapy

Unfractionated heparin and low molecular weight heparin
Unfractionated heparin is a heterogeneous mucopolysaccharide that binds antithrombin, which greatly potentiates the inhibition of thrombin and factor Xa.

An important limitation of unfractionated heparin is its unpredictable anticoagulant effect due to variable, non-specific binding to plasma proteins. Side effects include haemorrhage at the access site and heparin induced thrombocytopenia. About 10-20% of patients may develop type I thrombocytopenia, which is usually mild and self limiting. However, 0.3-3.0% of patients exposed to heparin for longer than five days develop the more serious immune mediated, type II thrombocytopenia, which paradoxically promotes thrombosis by platelet activation.

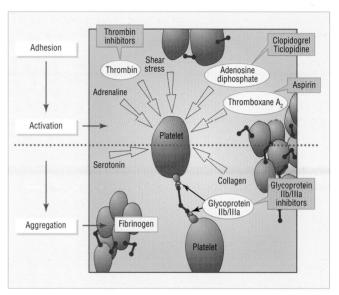

Action of antiplatelet and antithrombotic agents in inhibiting arterial thrombosis

---

Adjunctive pharmacology during percutaneous coronary intervention

Aspirin—For all clinical settings
Clopidogrel—For stenting; unstable angina or non-ST segment elevation myocardial infarction
Unfractionated heparin—For all clinical settings

Glycoprotein IIb/IIIa receptor inhibitors
Abciximab—For elective percutaneous intervention for chronic stable angina; unstable angina or non-ST segment elevation myocardial infarction (before and during percutaneous intervention); ST segment elevation myocardial infarction (before and during primary percutaneous intervention)
Eptifibatide—For elective percutaneous intervention for chronic stable angina; unstable angina or non-ST segment elevation myocardial infarction (before and during percutaneous intervention)
Tirofiban—For unstable angina or non-ST segment elevation myocardial infarction (before and during percutaneous intervention)

Comparison of unfractionated heparin and low molecular weight heparin

Unfractionated heparin	Low molecular weight heparin
Molecular weight—3000-30 000 Da	*Molecular weight*—4000-6000 Da
Mechanism of action—Binds antithrombin and inactivates factor Xa and thrombin equally (1:1)	*Mechanism of action*—Binds antithrombin and inactivates factor Xa more than thrombin (2-4:1)
Pharmacokinetics—Variable binding to plasma proteins, endothelial cells, and macrophages, giving unpredictable anticoagulant effects	*Pharmacokinetics*—Minimal plasma protein binding and no binding to endothelial cells and macrophages, giving predictable anticoagulant effects
Short half life	Longer half life
Reversible with protamine	Partially reversible with protamine
Laboratory monitoring—Activated clotting time	*Laboratory monitoring*—Not required
Cost—Inexpensive	*Cost*—10-20 times more expensive than unfractionated heparin

Despite these disadvantages, unfractionated heparin is cheap, relatively reliable, and reversible, with a brief duration of anticoagulant effect that can be rapidly reversed by protamine. It remains the antithrombotic treatment of choice during percutaneous coronary intervention.

For patients already taking a low molecular weight heparin who require urgent revascularisation, a switch to unfractionated heparin is generally recommended. Low molecular weight heparin is longer acting and only partially reversible with protamine. The use of low molecular weight heparin during percutaneous intervention is undergoing evaluation.

Direct thrombin inhibitors

These include hirudin, bivalirudin, lepirudin, and argatroban. They directly bind thrombin and act independently of antithrombin III. They bind less to plasma proteins and have a more predictable dose response than unfractionated heparin. At present, these drugs are used in patients with immune mediated heparin induced thrombocytopenia, but their potential for routine use during percutaneous intervention is being evaluated, in particular bivalirudin.

Antiplatelet drugs

Aspirin

Aspirin irreversibly inhibits cyclo-oxygenase, preventing the synthesis of prothrombotic thromboxane-A2 during platelet activation. Aspirin given before percutaneous intervention reduces the risk of abrupt arterial closure by 50-75%. It is well tolerated, with a low incidence of serious adverse effects. The standard dose results in full effect within hours, and in patients with established coronary artery disease it is given indefinitely. However, aspirin is only a mild antiplatelet agent and has no apparent effect in 10% of patients. These drawbacks have led to the development of another class of antiplatelet drugs, the thienopyridines.

Thienopyridines

Ticlopidine and clopidogrel irreversibly inhibit binding of adenosine diphosphate (ADP) during platelet activation. The combination of aspirin plus clopidogrel or ticlopidine has become standard antiplatelet treatment during stenting in order to prevent thrombosis within the stent. As clopidogrel has fewer serious side effects, a more rapid onset, and longer duration of action, it has largely replaced ticlopidine. The loading dose is 300 mg at the time of stenting or 75 mg daily for three days beforehand. It is continued for about four weeks, until new endothelium covers the inside of the stent. However, the recent CREDO study supports the much longer term (1 year) use of clopidogrel and aspirin after percutaneous coronary intervention, having found a significant (27%) reduction in combined risk of death, myocardial infarction, or stroke.

Glycoprotein IIb/IIIa receptor inhibitors

These are potent inhibitors of platelet aggregation. The three drugs in clinical use are abciximab, eptifibatide, and tirofiban. In combination with aspirin, clopidogrel (if a stent is to be deployed), and unfractionated heparin, they further decrease ischaemic complications in percutaneous coronary procedures.

Glycoprotein IIb/IIIa receptor inhibition may be beneficial in elective percutaneous intervention for chronic stable angina; for unstable angina or non-ST segment elevation myocardial infarction, for acute myocardial infarction with ST segment elevation.

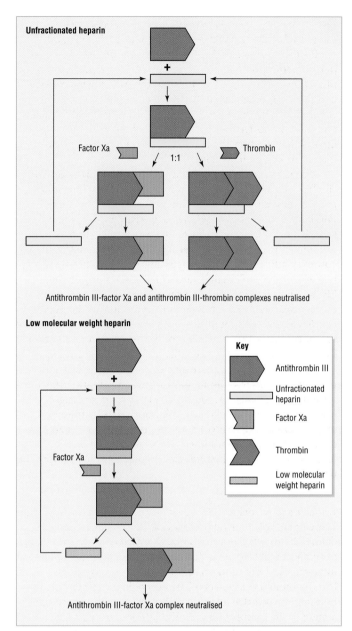

Mechanisms of catalytic inhibitory action of unfractionated heparin and low molecular weight heparin. Unfractionated heparin interacts with antithrombin III, accelerating binding and neutralisation of thrombin and factor Xa (in 1:1 ratio). Dissociated heparin is then free to re-bind with antithrombin III. Low molecular weight heparin is less able to bind thrombin because of its shorter length. This results in selective inactivation of factor Xa relative to thrombin. Irreversibly bound antithrombin III and factor Xa complex is neutralised, and dissociated low molecular weight heparin is free to re-bind with antithrombin III

Glycoprotein IIb/IIIa inhibitors currently in use

	Abciximab	Eptifibatide	Tirofiban
Source	Chimeric monoclonal mouse antibody	Peptide	Non-peptide
Time for platelet inhibition to return to normal (hours)	24-48	4-6	4-8
Approximate cost per percutaneous coronary intervention	$1031, €1023, £657 (12 hour infusion)	$263, €260, £167 (18 hour infusion)	$404, €401, £257 (18 hour infusion)
Severe thrombocytopenia	1.0% (higher if readministered)	Similar to placebo	Similar to placebo
Reversible with platelet transfusion?	Yes	No	No

Elective percutaneous intervention for chronic stable angina
Large trials have established the benefit of abciximab and eptifibatide during stenting for elective and urgent percutaneous procedures. As well as reducing risk of myocardial infarction during the procedure and the need for urgent repeat percutaneous intervention by 35-50%, these drugs seem to reduce mortality at one year (from 2.4% to 1% in EPISTENT and from 2% to 1.4% in ESPRIT). In diabetic patients undergoing stenting, the risk of complications was reduced to that of non-diabetic patients.

Although most trials showing the benefits of glycoprotein IIb/IIIa inhibitors during percutaneous coronary intervention relate to abciximab, many operators use the less expensive eptifibatide and tirofiban. However, abciximab seems to be superior to tirofiban, with lower 30 day mortality and rates of non-fatal myocardial infarction and urgent repeat percutaneous coronary intervention or coronary artery bypass graft surgery in a wide variety of circumstances (TARGET study). In the ESPRIT trial eptifibatide was primarily beneficial in stenting for elective percutaneous intervention, significantly reducing the combined end point of death, myocardial infarction, and urgent repeat percutaneous procedure or bypass surgery at 48 hours from 9.4% to 6.0%. These benefits were maintained at follow up.

As complication rates are already low during elective percutaneous intervention and glycoprotein IIb/IIIa inhibitors are expensive, many interventionists reserve these drugs for higher risk lesions or when complications occur. However, this may be misguided; ESPRIT showed that eptifibatide started at the time of percutaneous intervention was superior to a glycoprotein IIb/IIIa inhibitor started only when complications occurred.

Unstable angina and non-ST segment elevation myocardial infarction
The current role of glycoprotein IIb/IIIa inhibitors has been defined by results from several randomised trials. In one group of studies 29 885 patients (largely treated without percutaneous intervention) were randomised to receive a glycoprotein IIb/IIIa inhibitor or placebo. The end point of "30 day death or non-fatal myocardial infarction" showed an overall significant benefit of the glycoprotein IIb/IIIa inhibitor over placebo. Surprisingly, the largest trial (GUSTO IV ACS) showed no benefit with abciximab, which may be partly due to inclusion of lower risk patients. The use of glycoprotein IIb/IIIa inhibitors in all patients with unstable angina and non-ST segment elevation myocardial infarction remains debatable, although the consistent benefit seen with these drugs has led to the recommendation that they be given to high risk patients scheduled for percutaneous coronary intervention.

Another study (CURE) showed that the use of clopidogrel rather than a glycoprotein IIb/IIIa inhibitor significantly reduced the combined end point of cardiovascular death, non-fatal myocardial infarction, or stroke (from 11.4% to 9.3%). Similar benefits were seen in the subset of patients who underwent percutaneous coronary intervention. The impact this study will have on the use of glycoprotein IIb/IIIa inhibitors in this clinical situation remains unclear.

In another group of studies (n=16 770), patients were given a glycoprotein IIb/IIIa inhibitor or placebo immediately before or during planned percutaneous intervention. All showed unequivocal benefit with the active drug. Despite their efficacy, however, some interventionists are reluctant to use glycoprotein IIb/IIIa inhibitors in all patients because of their high costs and reserve their use for high risk lesions or when complications occur.

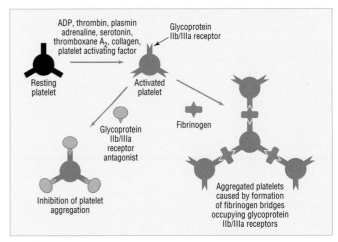

Mechanisms of activated platelet aggregation by fibrin cross linking and its blockade with glycoprotein IIb/IIIa inhibitors

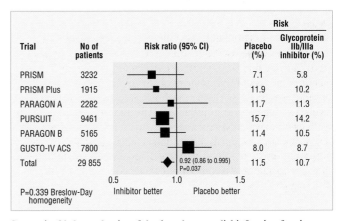

Composite 30 day end point of death and myocardial infarction for six medical treatment trials of glycoprotein IIb/IIIa inhibitors in unstable angina and non-ST segment elevation myocardial infarction

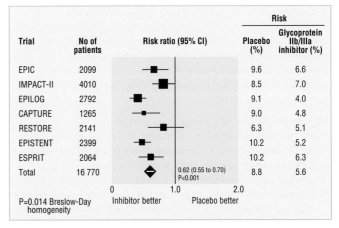

Composite 30 day end point of death and myocardial infarction for seven trials of glycoprotein IIb/IIIa inhibitors given before or during planned percutaneous coronary intervention for unstable angina and non-ST segment elevation myocardial infarction

Acute ST segment elevation myocardial infarction
In many centres primary percutaneous intervention is the preferred method of revascularisation for acute myocardial infarction. To date, randomised studies have shown that abciximab is the only drug to demonstrate benefit in this setting. The development of low cost alternatives and the potential for combination with other inhibitors of the coagulation cascade may increase the use of glycoprotein IIb/IIIa inhibitors.

Restenosis

Although coronary stents reduce restenosis rates compared with balloon angioplasty alone, restenosis within stents remains a problem. Nearly all systemic drugs aimed at reducing restenosis have failed, and drug eluting (coated) stents may ultimately provide the solution to this problem.

The future

Improvements in adjunctive pharmacotherapy, in combination with changes in device technology, will allow percutaneous coronary intervention to be performed with increased likelihood of acute and long term success and with lower procedural risks in a wider variety of clinical situations. Further refinements in antiplatelet treatment may soon occur with rapidly available bedside assays of platelet aggregation.

Competing interests: None declared.

Names of trials

- CAPTURE—C7E3 antiplatelet therapy in unstable refractory angina
- CREDO—Clopidogrel for the reduction of events during observation
- CURE—Clopidogrel in unstable angina to prevent recurrent events
- EPIC—Evaluation of C7E3 for prevention of ischemic complications
- EPILOG—Evaluation in PTCA to improve long-term outcome with abciximab glycoprotein IIb/IIIa blockade
- EPISTENT—Evaluation of IIb/IIIa platelet inhibitor for stenting
- ESPRIT—Enhanced suppression of the platelet glycoprotein IIb/IIIa receptor using integrilin therapy
- GUSTO IV-ACS—Global use of strategies to open occluded arteries IV in acute coronary syndrome
- IMPACT II—Integrilin to minimize platelet aggregation and coronary thrombosis
- PARAGON—Platelet IIb/IIIa antagonism for the reduction of acute coronary syndrome events in the global organization network
- PRISM—Platelet receptor inhibition in ischemic syndrome management
- PRISM-PLUS—Platelet receptor inhibition in ischemic syndrome management in patients limited by unstable signs and symptoms
- PURSUIT—Platelet glycoprotein IIb/IIIa in unstable angina: receptor suppression using integrilin therapy
- RESTORE—Randomized efficacy study of tirofiban for outcomes and restenosis

Further reading

- Lincoff AM, Califf RM, Moliterno DJ, Ellis SG, Ducas J, Kramer JH, et al. Complementary clinical benefits of coronary-artery stenting and blockade and blockade of platelet glycoprotein IIb/IIIa receptors. *N Engl J Med* 1999;341:319-27
- PURSUIT Trial Investigators. Inhibition of platelet glycoprotein IIb/IIIa with eptifibatide in patients with acute coronary syndromes. Platelet glycoprotein IIb/IIIa in unstable angina: receptor suppression using integrilin therapy. *N Engl J Med* 1998;339:436-43
- PRISM-PLUS Study Investigators. Inhibition of the platelet glycoprotein IIb/IIIa receptor with tirofiban in unstable angina and non-Q wave myocardial infarction. Platelet receptor inhibition in ischemic syndrome management in patients limited by unstable signs and symptoms. *N Engl J Med* 1998;338:1488-97
- ESPRIT Investigators. Novel dosing regimen of eptifibatide in planned coronary stent implantation (ESPRIT): a randomized, placebo-controlled trial. *Lancet* 2000;356:2037-44
- Boersma E, Harrington RA, Moliterno DJ, White H, Theroux P, Van de Werf F, et al. Platelet glycoprotein IIb/IIIa inhibitors in acute coronary syndromes: a meta-analysis of all major randomized clinical trials. *Lancet* 2002;359:189-98
- Chew DP, Lincoff AM. Adjunctive pharmacotherapy and coronary intervention. In: Grech ED, Ramsdale DR, eds. *Practical interventional cardiology*. 2nd ed. London: Martin Dunitz, 2002:207-24
- Steinhubl SR, Berger PB, Mann JT 3rd, Fry ET, DeLago A, Wilmer C, et al. Early and sustained dual oral antiplatelet therapy following percutaneous coronary intervention. A randomized controlled trial. *JAMA* 2002;288:2411-20

9 Non-coronary percutaneous intervention

Ever D Grech

Although most percutaneous interventional procedures involve the coronary arteries, major developments in non-coronary transcatheter cardiac procedures have occurred in the past 20 years. In adults the commonest procedures are balloon mitral valvuloplasty, ethanol septal ablation, and septal defect closure. These problems were once treatable only by surgery, but selected patients may now be offered less invasive alternatives. Carrying out such transcatheter procedures requires supplementary training to that for coronary intervention.

Balloon mitral valvuloplasty

Acquired mitral stenosis is a consequence of rheumatic fever and is commonest in developing countries. Commissural fusion, thickening, and calcification of the mitral valve leaflets typically occur, as well as thickening and shortening of the chordae tendinae. The mitral valve stenosis leads to left atrial enlargement, which predisposes patients to atrial fibrillation and the formation of left atrial thrombus.

In the 1980s percutaneous balloon valvuloplasty techniques were developed that could open the fused mitral commissures in a similar fashion to surgical commissurotomy. The resulting fall in pressure gradient and increase in mitral valve area led to symptomatic improvement. Today, this procedure is most often performed with the hourglass shaped Inoue balloon. This is introduced into the right atrium from the femoral vein, passed across the atrial septum by way of a septal puncture, and then positioned across the stenosed mitral valve before inflation.

Patient selection

In general, patients with moderate or severe mitral stenosis (valve area < 1.5 cm^2) with symptomatic disease despite optimal medical treatment can be considered for this procedure. Further patient selection relies heavily on transthoracic and transoesophageal echocardiographic findings, which provide structural information about the mitral valve and subvalvar apparatus.

A scoring system for predicting outcomes is commonly used to screen potential candidates. Four characteristics (valve mobility, leaflet thickening, subvalvar thickening, and calcification) are each graded 1 to 4. Patients with a score of ≤ 8 are more likely to have to have a good result than those with scores of > 8. Thus, patients with pliable, non-calcified valves and minimal fusion of the subvalvar apparatus achieve the best immediate and long term results.

Relative contraindications are the presence of pre-existing significant mitral regurgitation and left atrial thrombus. Successful balloon valvuloplasty increases valve area to > 1.5 cm^2 without a substantial increase in mitral regurgitation, resulting in significant symptomatic improvement.

Complications—The major procedural complications are death (1%), haemopericardium (usually during transseptal catheterisation) (1%), cerebrovascular embolisation (1%), severe mitral regurgitation (due to a torn valve cusp) (2%), and atrial septal defect (although this closes or decreases in size in most patients) (10%). Immediate and long term results are similar to those with surgical valvotomy, and balloon valvuloplasty can be repeated if commissural restenosis (a gradual process with an incidence of 30-40% at 6-8 years) occurs.

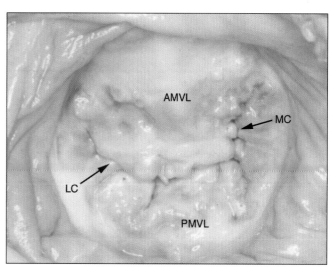

Stenotic mitral valve showing distorted, fused, and calcified valve leaflets. (AMVL=anterior mitral valve leaflet, PMVL=posterior mitral valve leaflet, LC=lateral commissure, MC=medial commissure)

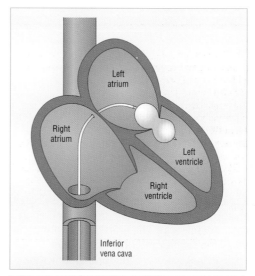

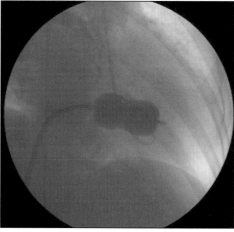

Top: Diagram of the Inoue balloon catheter positioned across a stenosed mitral valve. Bottom: Fluoroscopic image of the inflated Inoue balloon across the valve

In patients with suitable valvar anatomy, balloon valvuloplasty has become the treatment of choice for mitral stenosis, delaying the need for surgical intervention. It may also be of particular use in those patients who are at high risk of surgical intervention (because of pregnancy, age, or coexisting pulmonary or renal disease).

In contrast, balloon valvuloplasty for adult aortic stenosis is associated with high complication rates and poor outcomes and is only rarely performed.

Ethanol septal ablation

Hypertrophic cardiomyopathy

Hypertrophic cardiomyopathy is a disease of the myocytes caused by mutations in any one of 10 genes encoding various components of the sarcomeres. It is the commonest genetic cardiovascular disease, being inherited as an autosomal dominant trait and affecting about 1 in 500 of the population. It has highly variable clinical and pathological presentations.

It is usually diagnosed by echocardiography and is characterised by the presence of unexplained hypertrophy in a non-dilated left ventricle. In a quarter of cases septal enlargement may result in substantial obstruction of the left ventricular outflow tract. This is compounded by Venturi suction movement of the anterior mitral valve leaflet during ventricular systole, bringing it into contact with the hypertrophied septum. The systolic anterior motion of the anterior mitral valve leaflet also causes mitral regurgitation.

Treatment

Although hypertrophic cardiomyopathy is often asymptomatic, common symptoms are dyspnoea, angina, and exertional syncope, which may be related to the gradient in the left ventricular outflow tract. The aim of treatment of symptomatic patients is to improve functional disability, reduce the extent of obstruction of the left ventricular outflow tract, and improve diastolic filling. Treatments include negatively inotropic drugs such as β blockers, verapamil, and disopyramide. However, 10% of symptomatic patients fail to respond to drugs, and surgery—ventricular myectomy (which usually involves removal of a small amount of septal muscle) or ethanol septal ablation—can be considered.

The objective of ethanol septal ablation is to induce a localised septal myocardial infarction at the site of obstruction of the left ventricular outflow tract. The procedure involves threading a small balloon catheter into the septal artery supplying the culprit area of septum. Echocardiography with injection of an echocontrast agent down the septal artery allows the appropriate septal artery to be identified and reduces the number of unnecessary ethanol injections.

Once the appropriate artery is identified, the catheter balloon is inflated to completely occlude the vessel, and a small amount of dehydrated ethanol is injected through the central lumen of the catheter into the distal septal artery. This causes immediate vessel occlusion and localised myocardial infarction. The infarct reduces septal motion and thickness, enlarges the left ventricular outflow tract, and may decrease mitral valve systolic anterior motion, with consequent reduction in the gradient of the left ventricular outflow tract. Over the next few months the infarcted septum undergoes fibrosis and shrinkage, which may result in further symptomatic improvement.

The procedure is performed under local anaesthesia with sedation as required. Patients inevitably experience chest discomfort during ethanol injection, and treatment with intravenous opiate analgesics is essential. Patients are usually discharged after four or five days.

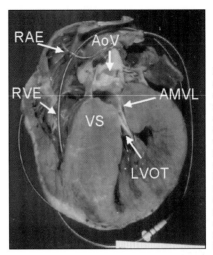

Postmortem appearance of a heart with hypertrophic cardiomyopathy showing massive ventricular and septal hypertrophy causing obstruction of the left ventricular outflow tract (LVOT). This is compounded by the anterior mitral valve leaflet (AMVL), which presses against the ventricular septum (VS). Note the coincidental right atrial (RAE) and right ventricular (RVE) pacing electrodes

Characteristics of hypertrophic cardiomyopathy

Anatomical—Ventricular hypertrophy of unknown cause, usually with disproportionate involvement of the interventricular septum
Physiological—Well preserved systolic ventricular function, impaired diastolic relaxation
Pathological—Extensive disarray and disorganisation of cardiac myocytes and increased interstitial collagen

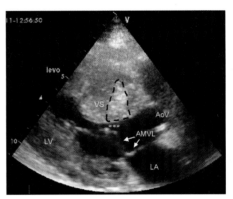

Echocardiogram showing anterior mitral valve leaflet (AMVL) and septal contact (***) during ventricular systole. Note marked left ventricular (LV) free wall and ventricular septal (VS) hypertrophy. Injection of an echocontrast agent down the septal artery results in an area of septal echo-brightness (dotted line). (LA=left atrium, AoV=aortic valve)

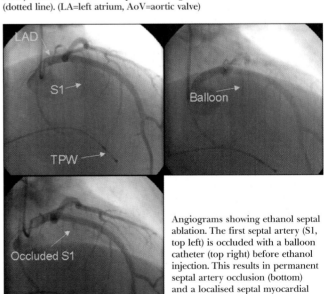

Angiograms showing ethanol septal ablation. The first septal artery (S1, top left) is occluded with a balloon catheter (top right) before ethanol injection. This results in permanent septal artery occlusion (bottom) and a localised septal myocardial infarction. (LAD=left anterior descending artery, TPW=temporary pacemaker wire)

Complications

Heart block is a frequent acute complication, so a temporary pacing electrode is inserted via the femoral vein beforehand and is usually left in situ for 24 hours after the procedure, during which time the patient is monitored.

The main procedural complications are persistent heart block requiring a permanent pacemaker (10%), coronary artery dissection and infarction requiring immediate coronary artery bypass grafting (2%), and death (1-2%). The procedural mortality and morbidity is similar to that for surgical myectomy, as is the reduction in left ventricular outflow tract gradient. Surgery and ethanol septal ablation have not as yet been directly compared in randomised studies.

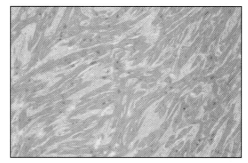

Micrograph of hypertrophied myocytes in haphazard alignments characteristic of hypertrophic cardiomyopathy. Interstitial collagen is also increased

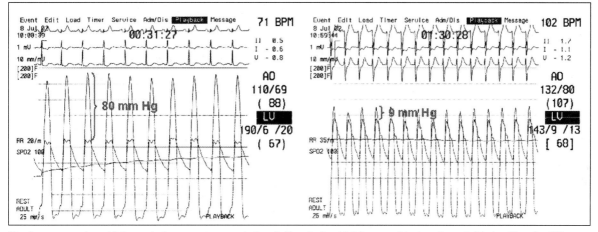

Simultaneous aortic and left ventricular pressure waves before (left) and after (right) successful ethanol septal ablation. Note the difference between left ventricular peak pressure and aortic peak pressure, which represents the left ventricular outflow tract gradient, has been reduced from 80 mm Hg to 9 mm Hg

Septal defect closure

Atrial septal defects

Atrial septal defects are congenital abnormalities characterised by a structural deficiency of the atrial septum and account for about 10% of all congenital cardiac disease. The commonest atrial septal defects affect the ostium secundum (in the fossa ovalis), and most are suitable for transcatheter closure. Although atrial septal defects may be closed in childhood, they are the commonest form of congenital heart disease to become apparent in adulthood.

Diagnosis is usually confirmed by echocardiography, allowing visualisation of the anatomy of the defect and Doppler estimation of the shunt size. The physiological importance of the defect depends on the duration and size of the shunt, as well as the response of the pulmonary vascular bed. Patients with significant shunts (defined as a ratio of pulmonary blood flow to systemic blood flow > 1.5) should be considered for closure when the diagnosis is made in later life because the defect reduces survival in adults who develop progressive pulmonary hypertension. They may also develop atrial tachyarrhythmias, which commonly precipitate heart failure.

Patients within certain parameters can be selected for transcatheter closure with a septal occluder. In those who are unsuitable for the procedure, surgical closure may be considered.

Patent foramen ovale

A patent foramen ovale is a persistent flap-like opening between the atrial septum primum and secundum which occurs in roughly 25% of adults. With microbubbles injected into a peripheral vein during echocardiography, a patent foramen ovale can be demonstrated by the patient performing and

Indications and contraindications for percutaneous closure of atrial septal defects

Indications

Clinical

- If defect causes symptoms
- Associated cerebrovascular embolic event
- Divers with neurological decompression sickness

- Pulmonary:systemic flow ratio > 1.5 and reversible pulmonary hypertension
- Right-to-left atrial shunt and hypoxaemia

Anatomical

- Defects within fossa ovalis (or patent foramen ovale)
- Defects with stretched diameter < 38 mm

- Presence of > 4 mm rim of tissue surrounding defect

Contraindications

- Sinus venosus defects
- Ostium primum defects

- Ostium secundum defects with other important congenital heart defects requiring surgical correction

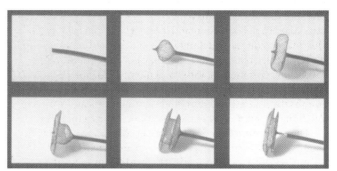

Deployment sequence of the Amplatzer septal occluder for closing an atrial septal defect

releasing a prolonged Valsalva manoeuvre. Visualisation of microbubbles crossing into the left atrium reveals a right-to-left shunt mediated by transient reversal of the interatrial pressure gradient.

Although a patent foramen ovale (or an atrial septal aneurysm) has no clinical importance in otherwise healthy adults, it may cause paradoxical embolism in patients with cryptogenic transient ischaemic attack or stroke (up to half of whom have a patent foramen ovale), decompression illness in divers, and right-to-left shunting in patients with right ventricular infarction or severe pulmonary hypertension. Patients with patent foramen ovale and paradoxical embolism have an approximate 3.5% yearly risk of recurrent cerebrovascular events.

Secondary preventive strategies are drug treatment (aspirin, clopidogrel, or warfarin), surgery, or percutaneous closure using a dedicated occluding device. A lack of randomised clinical trials directly comparing these options means optimal treatment remains uncertain. However, percutaneous closure offers a less invasive alternative to traditional surgery and allows patients to avoid potential side effects associated with anticoagulants and interactions with other drugs. In addition, divers taking anticoagulants may experience haemorrhage in the ear, sinus, or lung from barotrauma.

Congenital ventricular septal defects

Untreated congenital ventricular septal defects that require intervention are rare in adults. Recently, there has been interest in percutaneous device closure of ventricular septal defects acquired as a complication of acute myocardial infarction. However, more experience is necessary to assess the role of this procedure as a primary closure technique or as a bridge to subsequent surgery.

The picture of a stenotic mitral valve and micrograph of myocytes showing hypertrophic cardiomyopathy were provided by C Littman, consultant histopathologist at the Health Sciences Centre, Winnipeg, Manitoba, Canada. The postmortem picture of a heart with hypertrophic cardiomyopathy was provided by T Balachandra, chief medical examiner for the Province of Manitoba, Winnipeg. The pictures of Amplatzer occluder devices were provided by AGA Medical Corporation, Minnesota, USA.

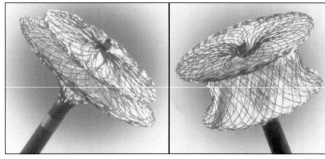

Amplatzer occluder devices for patent foramen ovale (left) and muscular ventricular septal defects (right)

Further reading

- Inoue K, Lau K-W, Hung J-S. Percutaneous transvenous mitral commissurotomy. In: Grech ED, Ramsdale DR, eds. *Practical interventional cardiology*. 2nd ed. London: Martin Dunitz, 2002: 373-87
- Bonow RO, Carabello B, de Leon AC, Edmunds LH Jr, Fedderly BJ, Freed MD, et al. ACC/AHA guidelines for the management of patients with valvular heart disease: A report of the American College of Cardiology/American Heart Association Task Force on Practice Guidelines (Committee on Management of Patients with Valvular Heart Disease). *J Am Coll Cardiol* 1998;32:1486-582
- Wilkins GT, Weyman AE, Abascal VM, Bloch PC, Palacios IF. Percutaneous balloon dilatation of the mitral valve: an analysis of echocardiographic variables related to outcome and the mechanism of dilatation. *Br Heart J* 1998;60:299-308
- Wigle ED, Rakowski H, Kimball BP, Williams WG. Hypertrophic cardiomyopathy: clinical spectrum and treatment. *Circulation* 1995; 92:1680-92
- Nagueh SF, Ommen SR, Lakkis NM, Killip D, Zoghbi WA, Schaff HV, et al. Comparison of ethanol septal reduction therapy with surgical myectomy for the treatment of hypertrophic obstructive cardiomyopathy. *J Am Coll Cardiol* 2001;38:1701-6
- Braun MU, Fassbender D, Schoen SP, Haass M, Schraeder R, Scholtz W, et al. Transcatheter closure of patent foramen ovale in patients with cerebral ischaemia. *J Am Coll Cardiol* 2002;39: 2019-25
- Waight DJ, Cao Q-L, Hijazi ZM. Interventional cardiac catheterisation in adults with congenital heart disease. In: Grech ED, Ramsdale DR, eds. *Practical interventional cardiology*. 2nd ed. London: Martin Dunitz, 2002:390-406

10 New developments in percutaneous coronary intervention

Julian Gunn, Ever D Grech, David Crossman, David Cumberland

Percutaneous coronary intervention has become a more common procedure than coronary artery bypass surgery in many countries, and the number of procedures continues to rise. In one day an interventionist may treat four to six patients with complex, multivessel disease or acute coronary syndromes. Various balloons, stents, and other devices are delivered by means of a 2 mm diameter catheter introduced via a peripheral artery. The success rate is over 95%, and the risk of serious complications is low. After a few hours patients can be mobilised, and they are usually discharged the same or the next day. Even the spectre of restenosis is now fading.

Refinements of existing techniques

The present success of percutaneous procedures is largely because of refinement of our "basic tools" (intracoronary guidewires and low profile balloons), which have greatly contributed to the safety and effectiveness of procedures. However, the greatest technological advance has been in the development of stents. These are usually cut by laser from stainless steel tubes into a variety of designs, each with different radial strength and flexibility. They are chemically etched or electropolished to a fine finish and sometimes coated.

Digital angiography is a great advance over cine-based systems, and relatively benign contrast media have replaced the toxic media used in early angioplasty. Although magnetic resonance and computed tomographic imaging may become useful in the non-invasive diagnosis of coronary artery disease, angiography will remain indispensable to guide percutaneous interventions for the foreseeable future.

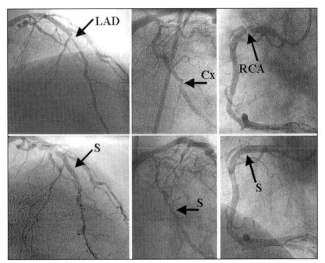

Triple vessel disease is no longer a surgical preserve, and particularly good results are expected with drug eluting stents. In this case, lesions in the left anterior descending (LAD), circumflex (Cx), and right coronary arteries (RCA) (top row) are treated easily and rapidly by stent (S) implantation (bottom row)

Interventional devices and their uses

Device	Use (% of cases)	Types of lesion
Balloon catheter	100%	Multiple types
Stent	70-90%	Most types
Drug eluting stent	0-50%	High risk of restenosis (possibly all)
Cutting balloon	1-5%	In-stent restenosis, ostial lesions
Rotablator	1-3%	Calcified, ostial, undilatable lesions
Brachytherapy	1-3%	In-stent restenosis
Atherectomy	<1%	Bulky, eccentric, ostial lesions
Stent graft	<1%	Aneurysm, arteriovenous malformation, perforation
Thrombectomy	<1%	Visible thrombus
Laser	<1%	Occlusions, in-stent restenosis
Distal protection	<1%	Degenerate vein graft

New device technology

Pre-eminent among new devices is the drug eluting (coated) stent, which acts as a drug delivery device to reduce restenosis. The first of these was the sirolimus coated Cypher stent.

Performance of percutaneous coronary intervention

General statistics

• Success rate of procedure	>95%
• Symptoms improved after procedure	90%
• Complications*	2%
• Restenosis	15% (range 5-50%)
• Duration of procedure	15 minutes-3 hours
• Access point:	
Femoral artery	95%
Radial or brachial artery	5%
• Time in hospital after procedure:	
Overnight	60%
Day case	20%
Longer	20%
• Intravenous contrast load	100-800 ml
• X ray dose to patient	75 Gy/cm²†

Special conditions

• Success of direct procedure for acute myocardial infarction	>95%
• Success for chronic (>3 month) occluded vessel	50-75%
• Mortality for procedure in severe cardiogenic shock	50%
• Restenosis:	
Vessels <2.5 mm in diameter, >40 mm length	60%
Vessels >3.5 mm diameter, <10 mm length	5%
• Lesion recurrence later than 6 months after procedure	<5%
• Re-restenosis:	
After repeat balloon dilatation	30-50%
After brachytherapy	<15%

*Death, myocardial infarction, coronary artery bypass surgery, cerebrovascular accident
†Equivalent to 1-2 computed tomography scans

Sirolimus is one of several agents that have powerful antimitotic effects and inhibit new tissue growth inside the artery and stent. In a randomised controlled trial (RAVEL) this stent gave a six month restenosis rate of 0% compared with 27% for an uncoated stent of the same design. A later randomised study (SIRIUS) of more complex stenoses (which are more prone to recur) still produced a low rate of restenosis within stented segments (9% v 36% with uncoated stents), even in patients with diabetes (18% v 51% respectively). Other randomised studies such as ASPECT and TAXUS II have also shown that coated stents (with the cytotoxic agent paclitaxel) have significantly lower six month restenosis rates than identical uncoated stents (14% v 39% and 6% v 20% respectively). By reducing the incidence of restenosis (and therefore recurrent symptoms), drug eluting stents will probably alter the balance of treating coronary artery disease in favour of percutaneous intervention rather than coronary artery bypass surgery. However, coated stents will not make any difference to the potential for percutaneous coronary intervention to achieve acute success in any given lesion; nor do they seem to have any impact on acute and subacute safety.

Although coated stents may, paradoxically, be too effective at altering the cellular response and thus delay the desirable process of re-endothelialisation, there is no evidence that this is a clinical problem. However, this problem has been observed with brachytherapy (catheter delivered radiotherapy over a short distance to kill dividing cells), a procedure that is generally reserved for cases of in-stent restenosis. This may lead to late thrombosis as platelets readily adhere to the "raw" surface that results from an impaired healing response. This risk is minimised by prolonged treatment with antiplatelet drugs and avoiding implanting any fresh stents at the time of brachytherapy.

Other energy sources may also prove useful. Sonotherapy (ultrasound) may have potential, less as a treatment in its own right than as a facilitator for gene delivery, and is "benign" in its effect on healthy tissue. Photodynamic therapy (the interaction of photosensitising drug, light, and tissue oxygen) is also being investigated but is still in early development. Laser energy, when delivered via a fine intracoronary wire, is used in a few centres to recanalise blocked arteries.

New work practices

Twenty years ago, a typical angioplasty treated one proximally located lesion in a single vessel in a patient with good left ventricular function. Now, it commonly treats two or three vessel disease, perhaps with multiple lesions (some of which may be complex), in patients with impaired left ventricular function, advanced age, and comorbidity. Patients may have undergone

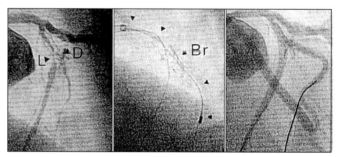

Angiograms showing severe, diffuse, in-stent restenosis in the left anterior descending artery and its diagonal branch (L and D, left). This was treated with balloon dilatation and brachytherapy with β irradiation (Novoste) from a catheter (Br, centre), with an excellent final result (right)

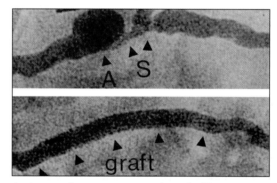

Angiogram of an aortocoronary vein graft with an aneurysm and stenoses (A and S, top). Treatment by implantation of a membrane-covered stent excluded the aneurysm and restored a tubular lumen (bottom)

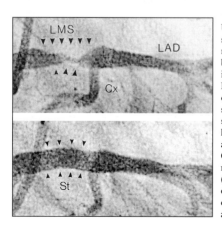

Unprotected left main stem stenoses (LMS, top) may, with careful selection, be treated by stent implantation (S, bottom). Best results (similar to coronary artery bypass surgery) are achieved in stable patients with good left ventricular function and no other disease. Close follow up to detect restenosis is important. (LAD=left anterior descending artery, Cx= circumflex coronary artery)

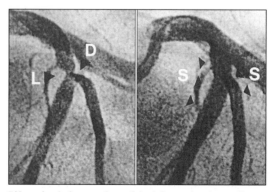

Bifurcation lesions, such as of the left anterior descending artery and its diagonal branch (L and D, left), are technically challenging to treat but can be well dilated by balloon dilatation and selective stenting (S, right)

coronary artery bypass surgery and be unsuitable for further heart surgery. Isolated left main stem and ostial right coronary artery lesions, though requiring more experience and variations on traditional techniques, are also no longer a surgical preserve.

Role of percutaneous coronary intervention

The role of percutaneous intervention has extended to the point where up to 70% of patients treated have acute coronary syndromes. Trial data now support the use of a combination of a glycoprotein IIb/IIIa inhibitor and early percutaneous intervention to give high risk patients the best long term results. The same applies to acute myocardial infarction, where percutaneous procedures achieve a much higher rate of arterial patency than thrombolytic treatment. Even cardiogenic shock, the most lethal of conditions, may be treated by an aggressive combination of intra-aortic balloon pumping and percutaneous intervention.

The potential for percutaneous procedures to treat a wide range of lesions successfully with low rates of restenosis raises the question of the relative roles of percutaneous intervention and bypass surgery in everyday practice. It takes time to accumulate sufficient trial data to make long term generalisations possible.

Early trials comparing balloon angioplasty with bypass surgery rarely included stents and few patients with three vessel disease (as such disease carried higher risk and percutaneous intervention was not as widely practised as now). The long term results favoured bypass surgery, but theses trials are now outdated. In the second generation of studies, stents were used in percutaneous intervention, improving the results. As in the early studies, surgery and intervention had similarly low complications and mortality. The intervention patients still had more need for repeat procedures because of restenosis than the bypass surgery patients, but the differences were less.

The major drawback of all these studies was an exclusion rate approaching 95%, making the general clinical application of the findings questionable. This was because it was unusual at that time to find patients with multivessel disease who were technically suitable for both methods and thus eligible for inclusion in the trials. Now that drug eluting stents are available, more trials are under way: the balance will now probably tip in favour of percutaneous coronary intervention. Meanwhile, the decision of which treatment is better for a patient at a given time is based on several factors, including the feasibility of percutaneous intervention (which is generally considered as the first option), completeness of revascularisation, comorbidity, age, and the patient's own preferences.

Implications for health services

These issues are likely to pose major problems for health services. Modern percutaneous techniques can be used both to shorten patients' stay in hospital and to make their treatment minimally hazardous and more comfortable. They can also be used in the first and the last (after coronary artery bypass surgery) stages of a patient's "ischaemic career."

On the other hand, for the role of percutaneous coronary intervention in acute infarction to be realised, universal emergency access to this service will be needed. However, most health systems cannot afford this—the main limiting factor being the number of interventionists and supporting staff required to allow a 24 hour rota compatible with legal working hours and the survival of routine elective work.

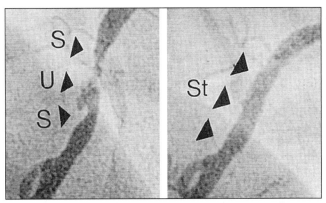

An acute coronary syndrome was found to be due to stenoses and an ulcerated plaque in the right coronary artery (S and U, left). This was treated with a glycoprotein IIb/IIIa inhibitor followed by stent implantation (right). This is an increasingly common presentation of coronary artery disease to catheterisation laboratories

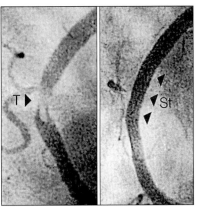

Right coronary artery containing large, lobulated thrombus (T, left) on a substantial stenosis. After treatment with glycoprotein IIb/IIIa inhibitor, the lesion was stented successfully (St, right)

General roles of percutaneous coronary intervention (PCI) and coronary artery bypass surgery (CABG)

Condition	PCI		CABG
	1993	2003	
Acute presentation			
Acute coronary syndrome	++	+++	++
Cardiogenic shock	+/−	+	+/−
Acute full thickness myocardial infarction	+	+++	−
Bailout after failed thrombolysis	+	++	−
Chronic presentation			
Impaired left ventricle with left main stem stenosis and blocked right coronary artery	− −	−	+++
Impaired left ventricle and 3 vessel disease	+	++	+++
Impaired left ventricle and 3 vessel disease with ≥ 1 occlusion	−	+	+++
Diabetes and 3 vessel disease	+	++	+++
Good left ventricle and 3 vessel disease	+	++	+++
2 occluded vessels	−	−	++
Good left ventricle and 2 vessel disease	+	+++	++
Repeat revascularisation after PCI	++	+++	++
Good left ventricle and 1 vessel disease	+++	+++	+
2-3 vessel diffuse or distal disease	+	++	+
Repeat revascularisation after CABG	+	++	+
Palliative partial revascularisation	+	++	−
Revascularisation of frail patient or with severe comorbidity	+	++	−

+++ highly effective role, ++ useful role, + limited role, − treatment not preferred, − − treatment usually strongly advised against

The future for percutaneous coronary intervention

Will percutaneous coronary intervention exist in 20 years time, or, at least, be recognisable as a logical development of today's procedures? Will balloons and stents still be in use? It is likely that percutaneous procedures will expand further, although some form of biodegradable stent is a possibility. A more "biological" stent might also be able to act as an effective drug or gene reservoir, which may extend local drug delivery into new areas of coronary artery disease. We may find ourselves detecting inflamed ("hot") plaques with thermography catheters and treating these before they rupture. We may even be able to modify the natural course of coronary artery disease by releasing agents "remotely" (possibly using an external ultrasound trigger) or by injecting an agent that activates the molecular cargo in a stent.

A persistent challenge still limiting the use of percutaneous coronary intervention is that of chronic total occlusions, which can be too tough to allow passage of an angioplasty guidewire. An intriguing technique is percutaneous in situ coronary artery bypass. With skill and ingenuity, a few enthusiasts have anastomosed the stump of a blocked coronary artery to the adjacent cardiac vein under intracoronary ultrasound guidance, thereby using the vein as an endogenous conduit (with reversed flow). This technique may assist only a minority of patients. More practical, we believe, is the concept of drilling through occlusions with some form of external guidance, perhaps magnetic fields.

"Direct" myocardial revascularisation (punching an array of holes into ischaemic myocardium) has had a mixed press over the past decade. Some attribute its effect to new vessel formation, others cite a placebo effect. Although the channels do not stay open, they seem to stimulate new microvessels to grow. Injection of growth factors (vascular endothelial growth factor and fibroblast growth factor) to induce new blood vessel growth also has this effect, and percutaneous injection of these agents into scarred or ischaemic myocardium is achievable. However, we need a more thorough understanding of biological control mechanisms before we can be confident of the benefits of this technology.

Challenges to mechanical revascularisation

Deaths from coronary artery disease are being steadily reduced in the Western world. However, with increasing longevity, it is unlikely that we will see a reduction in the prevalence of its chronic symptoms. More effective primary and secondary prevention; antismoking and healthy lifestyle campaigns; and the widespread use of antiplatelet drugs, β blockers, statins, and renin-angiotensin system inhibitors may help prevent, or at least delay, the presentation of symptomatic coronary artery disease. In patients undergoing revascularisation, they are essential components of the treatment "package." More effective anti-atherogenic treatments will no doubt emerge in the near future to complement and challenge the dramatic progress being made in percutaneous coronary intervention.

Further reading

- Morice M-C, Serruys PW, Sousa JE, Fajadet J, Ban Hayashi E, Perin M, et al. A randomized comparison of a sirolimus-eluting stent with a standard stent for coronary revascularization. *N Engl J Med* 2002;346:1773-80
- Park SJ, Shim WH, Ho DS, Raizner AE, Park SW, Hong MK, et al. A paclitaxel-eluting stent for the prevention of coronary restenosis. *N Engl J Med* 2003;348:1537-45
- Raco DL, Yusuf S. Overview of randomised trials of percutaneous coronary intervention: comparison with medical and surgical therapy for chronic coronary artery disease. In: Grech ED, Ramsdale DR, eds. *Practical interventional cardiology.* 2nd ed. London: Martin Dunitz, 2002:263-77
- Teirstein PS, Kuntz RE. New frontiers in interventional cardiology: intravascular radiation to prevent restenosis. *Circulation* 2001;104: 2620-6
- Tsuji T, Tamai H, Igaki K, Kyo E, Kosuga K, Hata T, et al. Biodegradable stents as a platform to drug loading. *Int J Cardiovasc Intervent* 2003;5:13-6
- Hariawala MD, Sellke FW. Angiogenesis and the heart: therapeutic implications. *J R Soc Med* 1997;90:307-11
- Serruys PW, Unger F, Sousa JE, Jatene A, Bonnier HJ, Schonberger JP, et al, for the Arterial Revascularization Therapies Study Group. Comparison of coronary-artery bypass surgery and stenting for the treatment of multivessel disease. *N Engl J Med* 2001;344:1117-24
- SoS Investigators. Coronary artery bypass surgery versus percutaneous coronary intervention with stent implantation in patients with multivessel coronary artery disease (the stent or surgery trial): a randomised controlled trial. *Lancet* 2002;360: 965-70

The coronary artery imaging was provided by John Bowles, clinical specialist radiographer, and Nancy Alford, clinical photographer, Sheffield Teaching Hospitals NHS Trust, Sheffield.

Competing interests: None declared.

11 Percutaneous interventional electrophysiology

Gerry C Kaye

Before the 1980s, cardiac electrophysiology was primarily used to confirm mechanisms of arrhythmia, with management mainly by pharmacological means. However, recognised shortcomings in antiarrhythmic drugs spurred the development of non-pharmacological treatments, particularly radiofrequency ablation and implantable defibrillators.

The two major mechanisms by which arrhythmias occur are automaticity and re-entrant excitation. Most arrhythmias are of the re-entrant type and require two or more pathways that are anatomically or functionally distinct but in electrical contact. The conduction in one pathway must also be slowed to a sufficient degree to allow recovery of the other so that an electrical impulse may then re-enter the area of slowed conduction.

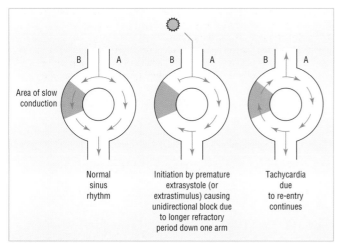

Mechanism of a re-entry circuit. An excitation wave is propagated at a normal rate down path A, but slowly down path B. An excitation wave from an extrasystole now encounters the slow pathway (B), which is still refractory, creating unidirectional block. There is now retrograde conduction from path A, which coincides with the end of the refractory period in path B. This gives rise to a persistent circus movement

Intracardiac electrophysiological studies

Intracardiac electrophysiological studies give valuable information about normal and abnormal electrophysiology of intracardiac structures. They are used to confirm the mechanism of an arrhythmia, to delineate its anatomical substrate, and to ablate it. The electrical stability of the ventricles can also be assessed, as can the effects of an antiarrhythmic regimen.

Atrioventricular conduction

Electrodes positioned at various sites in the heart can give only limited data about intracardiac conduction during sinus rhythm at rest. "Stressing" the system allows more information to be generated, particularly concerning atrioventricular nodal conduction and the presence of accessory pathways.

By convention, the atria are paced at 100 beats/min for eight beats. The ninth beat is premature (extrastimulus), and the AH interval (the time between the atrial signal (A) and the His signal (H), which represents atrioventricular node conduction

Classification of arrhythmias

Indications for electrophysiological studies

Investigation of symptoms
- History of persistent palpitations
- Recurrent syncope
- Presyncope with impaired left ventricular function

Interventions
- Radiofrequency ablation—Accessory pathways, junctional tachycardias, atrial flutter, atrial fibrillation
- Investigation of arrhythmias (narrow and broad complex) with or without radiofrequency ablation
- Assessment or ablation of ventricular arrhythmias

Contraindications
- Severe aortic stenosis, unstable coronary disease, left main stem stenosis, substantial electrolyte disturbance

---

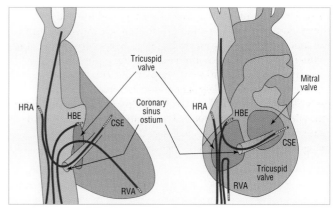

Diagrams showing position of pacing or recording electrodes in the heart in the right anterior oblique and left anterior oblique views (views from the right and left sides of the chest respectively). HRA=high right atrial electrode, usually on the lateral wall or appendage; HBE=His bundle electrode, on the medial aspect of the tricuspid valve; RVA=right ventricular apex; CSE=coronary sinus electrode, which records electrical deflections from the left side of the heart between the atrium and ventricle

time) is measured. This sequence is repeated with the ninth beat made increasingly premature. In normal atrioventricular nodal conduction, the AH interval gradually increases as the extrastimulus becomes more premature and is graphically represented as the atrioventricular nodal curve. The gradual prolongation of the AH interval (decremental conduction) is a feature that rarely occurs in accessory pathway conduction.

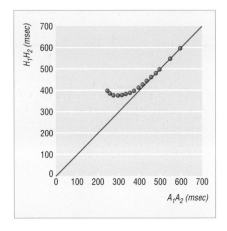

A normal atrioventricular nodal "hockey stick" curve during antegrade conduction of atrial extrastimuli. As the atrial extrastimulus (A_1-A_2) becomes more premature, the AH interval (H_1-H_2) shortens until the atrioventricular node becomes functionally refractory

Retrograde ventriculoatrial conduction

Retrograde conduction through the atrioventricular node is assessed by pacing the ventricle and observing conduction back into the atria. The coronary sinus electrode is critically important for this. It lies between the left ventricle and atrium and provides information about signals passing over the left side of the heart. The sequence of signals that pass from the ventricle to the atria is called the retrograde activation sequence.

If an accessory pathway is present, this sequence changes: with left sided pathways, there is an apparent "short circuit" in the coronary sinus with a shorter ventriculoatrial conduction time. This is termed a concealed pathway, as its effect cannot be seen on a surface electrocardiogram. It conducts retrogradely only, unlike in Wolff-Parkinson-White syndrome, where the pathway is bidirectional. Often intracardiac electrophysiological studies are the only way to diagnose concealed accessory pathways, which form the basis for many tachycardias with narrow QRS complexes.

Supraventricular tachycardia

Supraventricular tachycardias have narrow QRS complexes with rates between 150-250 beats/min. The two common mechanisms involve re-entry due to either an accessory pathway (overt as in Wolff-Parkinson-White syndrome or concealed) or junctional re-entry tachycardia.

Accessory pathways

These lie between the atria and ventricles in the atrioventricular ring, and most are left sided. Arrhythmias are usually initiated by an extrasystole or, during intracardiac electrophysiological studies, by an extrastimulus, either atrial or ventricular. The extrasystole produces delay within the atrioventricular node, allowing the signal, which has passed to the ventricle, to re-enter the atria via the accessory pathway. This may reach the atrioventricular node before the next sinus beat arrives but when the atrioventricular node is no longer refractory, thus allowing the impulse to pass down the His bundle and back up to the atrium through the pathway. As ventricular depolarisation is normal, QRS complexes are narrow. This circuit accounts for over 90% of supraventricular tachycardias in

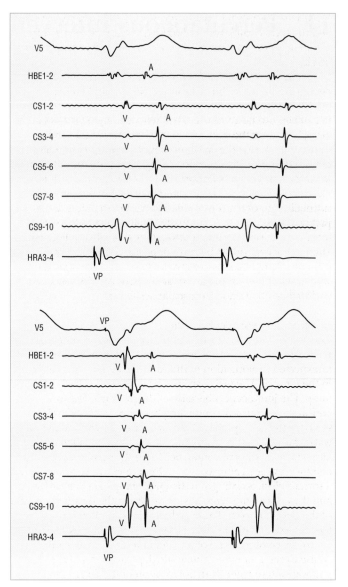

Coronary sinus electrode signals, with poles CS9-10 placed proximally near the origin of the coronary sinus and poles 1-2 placed distally reflecting changes in the left ventricular-left atrial free wall. Top: normal retrograde activation sequence with depolarisation passing from the ventricle back through the atrioventricular node to the right atrium and simultaneously across the coronary sinus to the left atrium. Bottom: retrograde activation sequence in the presence of an accessory pathway in the free wall of the left ventricle showing a shorter ventriculoatrial (VA) time than would be expected in the distal coronary sinus electrodes (CS1-2). Such a pathway would not be discernible from a surface electrocardiogram

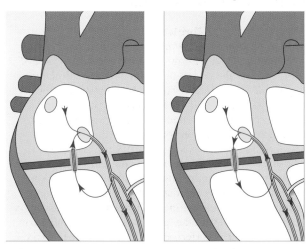

Mechanisms for orthodromic (left) and antedromic (right) atrioventricular re-entrant tachycardia

Wolff-Parkinson-White syndrome. Rarely, the circuit is reversed, and the QRS complexes are broad as the ventricles are fully pre-excited. This rhythm is often misdiagnosed as ventricular in origin.

Treatment—Pathway ablation effects a complete cure by destroying the arrhythmia substrate. Steerable ablation catheters allow most areas within the heart to be reached. The left atrium can be accessed either retrogradely via the aortic valve, by flexing the catheter tip through the mitral valve, or transseptally across the atrial septum. Radiofrequency energy is delivered to the atrial insertion of a pathway and usually results in either a rapid disappearance of pre-excitation on the surface electrocardiogram or, in the case of concealed pathways, normalisation of the retrograde activation sequence. Accessory pathway ablation is 95% successful. Failure occurs from an inability to accurately map pathways or difficulty in delivering enough energy, usually because of positional instability of the catheter. Complications are rare ($<0.5\%$) and are related to vascular access—femoral artery aneurysms or, with left sided pathways, embolic cerebrovascular accidents.

Junctional re-entry tachycardia

This is the commonest cause of paroxysmal supraventricular tachycardia. The atrioventricular nodal curve shows a sudden unexpected prolongation of the AH interval known as a "jump" in the interval. The tachycardia is initiated at or shortly after the jump. The jump occurs because of the presence of two pathways—one slowly conducting but with relatively rapid recovery (the slow pathway), the other rapidly conducting but with relatively slow recovery (the fast pathway)—called duality of atrioventricular nodal conduction. This disparity between conduction speed and recovery allows re-entrance to occur. On a surface electrocardiogram the QRS complexes are narrow, and the P waves are often absent or distort the terminal portion of the QRS complex. These arrhythmias can often be terminated by critically timed atrial or ventricular extrastimuli.

In the common type of junctional re-entry tachycardia (type A) the circuit comprises antegrade depolarisation of the slow pathway and retrograde depolarisation of the fast pathway. Rarely ($<5\%$ of junctional re-entry tachycardias) the circuit is reversed (type B). The slow and fast pathways are anatomically separate, with both inputting to an area called the compact atrioventricular node. The arrhythmia can be cured by mapping and ablating either the slow or fast pathway, and overall success occurs in 98% of cases. Irreversible complete heart block requiring a permanent pacemaker occurs in 1-2% of cases, with the risk being higher for fast pathway ablation. Therefore, slow pathway ablation is the more usual approach.

Atrial flutter and atrial fibrillation

Atrial flutter is a macro re-entrant circuit within the right atrium. The critical area of slow conduction lies at the base of the right atrium in the region of the slow atrioventricular nodal pathway. Producing a discrete line of ablation between the tricuspid annulus and the inferior vena cava gives a line of electrical block and is associated with a high success rate in terminating flutter. Flutter responds poorly to standard antiarrhythmic drugs, and ablation carries a sufficiently impressive success rate to make it a standard treatment.

Atrial fibrillation is caused by micro re-entrant wavelets circulating around the great venous structures, or it may be related to a focus of atrial ectopy arising within the pulmonary veins at their junction with the left atrium. The first indication that atrial fibrillation was electrically treatable came from the Maze operation (1990). Electrical dissociation of the atria from the great veins was carried out by surgical excision of the veins

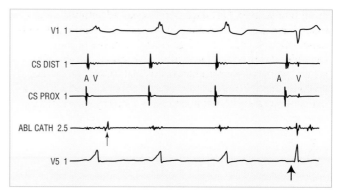

Surface electrocardiogram leads V1 and V5 and signals from the distal coronary sinus electrodes (CS dist), proximal electrodes (CS prox), and the tip of the ablation catheter (ABL CATH) during pathway ablation to treat Wolff-Parkinson-White syndrome. The onset of radiofrequency energy (thin arrow) produces loss of pre-excitation after two beats with a narrow complex QRS seen at the fourth beat (broad arrow). Prolongation of the AV signal in the coronary sinus occurs when pre-excitation is lost

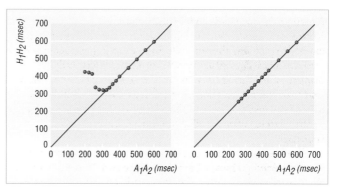

Atrioventricular nodal curves. In a patient with slow-fast junctional re-entrant tachycardia (left) there is a "jump" in atrioventricular nodal conduction when conduction changes from the fast to the slow pathway. In a patient with accessory pathways conducting antegradely (such as Wolff-Parkinson-White syndrome) there is no slowing of conduction as seen in the normal atrioventricular node, and the curve reflects conduction exclusively over the pathway (right)

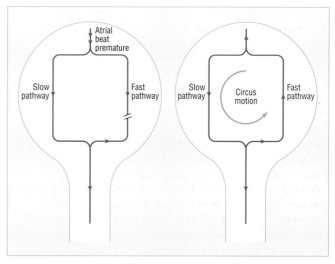

Mechanism of slow-fast junctional re-entrant tachycardia. A premature atrial impulse finds the fast pathway refractory, allowing retrograde conduction back up to the atria

from their insertion sites and then suturing them back. The scarred areas acted as insulation, preventing atrial wave-fronts from circulating within the atria. Similar lines of block can be achieved by catheter ablation within the right and left atria. The results look promising, although this is a difficult, prolonged procedure with a high relapse rate. Of more interest is a sub-group of patients with runs of atrial ectopy, which degenerate to paroxysms of atrial fibrillation. These extrasystoles usually originate from the pulmonary veins, and their ablation substantially reduces the frequency of symptomatic atrial fibrillation. With better understanding of the underlying mechanisms and improved techniques, atrial fibrillation may soon become a completely ablatable arrhythmia.

Ventricular tachycardia

Ventricular tachycardia carries a serious adverse prognosis, particularly in the presence of coronary artery disease and impaired ventricular function. Treatment options include drugs, occasional surgical intervention (bypass or arrhythmia surgery), and implantable defibrillators, either alone or in combination. Ventricular tachycardia can be broadly divided into two groups, ischaemic and non-ischaemic. The latter includes arrhythmias arising from the right ventricular outflow tract and those associated with cardiomyopathies.

Since the radiofrequency energy of an ablation catheter is destructive only at the site of the catheter tip, this approach lends itself more to arrhythmias where a discrete abnormality can be described, such as non-ischaemic ventricular tachycardia. In ischaemic ventricular tachycardia, where the abnormal substrate often occurs over a wide area, the success rate is lower.

Ideally, the arrhythmia should be haemodynamically stable, reliably initiated with ventricular pacing, and mapped to a localised area within the ventricle. In many cases, however, this is not possible. The arrhythmia may be unstable after initiation and therefore cannot be mapped accurately. The circuit may also lie deep within the ventricular wall and cannot be fully ablated. However, detailed intracardiac maps can be made with multipolar catheters. A newer approach is the use of a non-contact mapping catheter, which floats freely within the ventricles but senses myocardial electrical circuits.

Although the overall, long term, success rate for radiofrequency ablation of ischaemic ventricular tachycardia is only about 65%, this may increase.

Conclusion

The electrophysiological approach to treating arrhythmias has been revolutionised by radiofrequency ablation. Better computerised mapping, improved catheters, and more efficient energy delivery has enabled many arrhythmias to be treated and cured. The ability to ablate some forms of atrial fibrillation and improvement in ablation of ventricular tachycardia is heralding a new age of electrophysiology. Ten years ago it could have been said that electrophysiologists were a relatively benign breed of cardiologists who did little harm but little good either. That has emphatically changed, and it can now be attested that electrophysiologists exact the only true cure in cardiology.

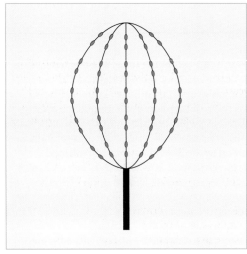

Diagram of basket-shaped mapping catheter with several recording electrodes (red dots). The basket retracts into a catheter for placement in either the atria or ventricles. Once it is in position, retraction of the catheter allows the basket to expand

Further reading

- Olgin JE, Zipes DP. Specific arrhythmias: diagnosis and treatment. In: Braunwald E, Zipes DP, Libby P, eds. *Heart disease*. 6th ed. Philadelphia: Saunders, 2001:1877-85
- McGuire MA, Janse MJ. New insights on the anatomical location of components of the reentrant circuit and ablation therapy for atrioventricular reentrant tachycardia. *Curr Opin Cardiol* 1995; 10:3-8
- Jackman WM, Beckman KJ, McClelland JH, Wang X, Friday KJ, Roman CA, et al. Treatment of supraventricular tachycardia due to atrioventricular nodal re-entry by radiofrequency catheter ablation of the slow-pathway conduction. *N Engl J Med* 1992;327:313-8
- Calkins H, Leon AR, Deam AG, Kalbfleisch SJ, Langberg JJ, Morady F. Catheter ablation of atrial flutter using radiofrequency energy. *Am J Cardiol* 1994;73:353-6
- Schilling RJ, Peter NS, Davies DW. Feasibility of a non-contact catheter for endocardial mapping of human ventricular tachycardia. *Circulation* 1999;99:2543-52

Competing interests: None declared.

The diagrams showing the mechanisms of orthodromic and antedromic atrioventricular re-entrant tachycardia and of slow-fast atrioventricular nodal re-entrant tachycardia are reproduced from *ABC of Clinical Electrocardiography*, edited by Francis Morris, 2002.

12 Implantable devices for treating tachyarrhythmias

Timothy Houghton, Gerry C Kaye

Pacing treatment for tachycardia control has achieved success, notably in supraventricular tachycardia. Pacing termination for ventricular tachycardia has been more challenging, but an understanding of arrhythmia mechanisms, combined with increasingly sophisticated pacemakers and the ability to deliver intracardiac pacing and shocks, have led to success with implantable cardioverter defibrillators.

Mechanisms of pacing termination

There are two methods of pace termination.

Underdrive pacing was used by early pacemakers to treat supraventricular and ventricular tachycardias. Extrastimuli are introduced at a constant interval, but at a slower rate than the tachycardia, until one arrives during a critical period, terminating the tachycardia. Because of the lack of sensing of the underlying tachycardia, there is a risk of a paced beat falling on the T wave, producing ventricular fibrillation or ventricular tachycardia, or degenerating supraventricular tachycardias to atrial fibrillation. It is also not particularly successful at terminating supraventricular tachycardia or ventricular tachycardia and is no longer used routinely.

Overdrive pacing is more effective for terminating both supraventricular and ventricular tachycardias. It is painless, quick, effective, and associated with low battery drain of the pacemaker. Implantation of devices for terminating supraventricular tachycardias is now rarely required because of the high success rate of radiofrequency ablative procedures (see previous article). Overdrive pacing for ventricular tachycardia is often successful but may cause acceleration or induce ventricular fibrillation. Therefore, any device capable of pace termination of ventricular tachycardia must also have defibrillatory capability.

Implantable cardioverter defibrillators

Initially, cardioverter defibrillator implantation was a major operation requiring thoracotomy and was associated with 3-5% mortality. The defibrillation electrodes were patches sewn on to the myocardium, and leads were tunnelled subcutaneously to the device, which was implanted in a subcutaneous abdominal pocket. Early devices were large and often shocked patients inappropriately, mainly because these relatively unsophisticated units could not distinguish ventricular tachycardia from supraventricular tachycardia.

Current implantation procedures

Modern implantable cardioverter defibrillators are transvenous systems, so no thoracotomy is required and implantation mortality is about 0.5%. The device is implanted either subcutaneously, as for a pacemaker, in the left or right deltopectoral area, or subpectorally in thin patients to prevent the device eroding the skin.

The ventricular lead tip is positioned in the right ventricular apex, and a second lead can be positioned in the right atrial appendage to allow dual chamber pacing if required and discrimination between atrial and ventricular tachycardias. The ventricular defibrillator lead has either one or two shocking coils. For two-coil leads, one is proximal (usually within the superior vena cava), and one is distal (right ventricular apex).

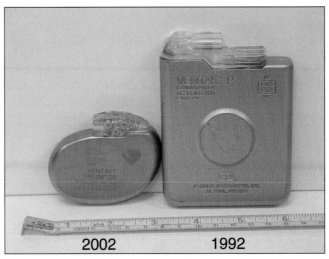

2002   1992

Changes in implantable cardioverter defibrillators over 10 years (1992-2002). Apart from the marked reduction in size, the implant technique and required hardware have also dramatically improved—from the sternotomy approach with four leads and abdominal implantation to the present two-lead transvenous endocardial approach that is no more invasive than a pacemaker implant

---

Mechanisms of arrhythmias

Unicellular	Multicellular
● Enhanced automaticity	● Re-entry
● Triggered activity—early or delayed after depolarisations	● Electrotonic interaction
	● Mechanico-electrical coupling

Arrhythmias associated with re-entry

- Atrial flutter
- Sinus node re-entry tachycardia
- Junctional re-entry tachycardia
- Atrioventricular reciprocating tachycardias (such as Wolff-Parkinson-White syndrome)
- Ventricular tachycardia

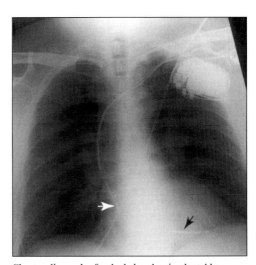

Chest radiograph of a dual chamber implantable cardioverter defibrillator with a dual coil ventricular lead (black arrow) and right atrial lead (white arrow)

During implantation the unit is tested under conscious sedation. Satisfactory sensing during sinus rhythm, ventricular tachycardia, and ventricular fibrillation is established, as well as pacing and defibrillatory thresholds. Defibrillatory thresholds should be at least 10 joules less then the maximum output of the defibrillator (about 30 joules).

New developments

An important development is the implantable cardioverter defibrillator's ability to record intracardiac electrograms. This allows monitoring of each episode of anti-tachycardia pacing or defibrillation. If treatment has been inappropriate, then programming changes can be made with a programming unit placed over the defibrillator site.

Current devices use anti-tachycardia pacing, with low and high energy shocks also available—known as tiered therapy. Anti-tachycardia pacing can take the form of adaptive burst pacing, with cycle length usually about 80-90% of that of the ventricular tachycardia. Pacing bursts can be fixed (constant cycle length) or autodecremental, when the pacing burst accelerates (each cycle length becomes shorter as the pacing train progresses). Should anti-tachycardia pacing fail, low energy shocks are given first to try to terminate ventricular tachycardia with the minimum of pain (as some patients remain conscious despite rapid ventricular tachycardia) and reduce battery drain, thereby increasing device longevity.

With the advent of dual chamber systems and improved diagnostic algorithms, shocking is mostly avoided during supraventricular tachycardia. Even in single lead systems the algorithms are now sufficiently sophisticated to differentiate between supraventricular tachycardia and ventricular tachycardia. There is a rate stability function, which assesses cycle length variability and helps to exclude atrial fibrillation.

Device recognition of tachyarrhythmias is based mainly on the tachycardia cycle length, which can initiate anti-tachycardia pacing or low energy or high energy shocks. With rapid tachycardias, the device can be programmed to give a high energy shock as first line treatment.

Complications

These include infection; perforation, displacement, fracture, or insulation breakdown of the leads; oversensing or undersensing of the arrhythmia; and inappropriate shocks for sinus tachycardia or supraventricular tachycardia. Psychological problems are common, and counselling plays an important role. Regular follow up is required. If antiarrhythmic drugs are taken the potential use of an implantable cardioverter defibrillator is reduced.

Precautions—after patient death the device must be switched off before removal otherwise a severe electric shock can be delivered to the person removing the device. The implanting centre or local hospital should be informed that the patient has died and arrangements can usually be made to turn the ICD off. The device must be removed before cremation.

Driving and implantable cardioverter defibrillators

The UK Driver and Vehicle Licensing Agency recommends that group 1 (private motor car) licence holders are prohibited from driving for six months after implantation of a defibrillator when there have been preceding symptoms of an arrhythmia. If a shock is delivered within this period, driving is withheld for a further six months.

Any change in device programming or antiarrhythmic drugs means a month of abstinence from driving, and all patients must remain under regular review. There is a five year prohibition on driving if treatment or the arrhythmia is associated with incapacity.

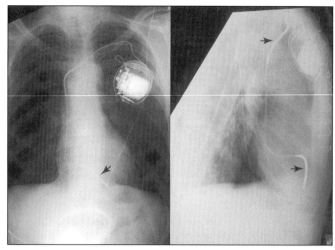

Posteroanterior and lateral chest radiographs of transvenous implantable cardioverter defibrillator showing the proximal and distal lead coils (arrows)

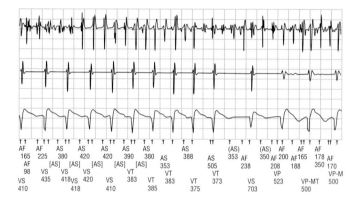

Intracardiac electrograms from an implantable cardioverter defibrillator. Upper recording is intra-atrial electrogram, which shows atrial fibrillation. Middle and lower tracings are intracardiac electrograms from ventricle

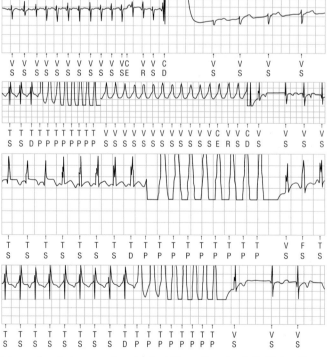

Intracardiac electrograms from implantable cardioverter defibrillators. Top: Ventricular tachycardia terminated with a single high energy shock. Second down: Ventricular tachycardia acceleration after unsuccessful ramp pacing, which was then terminated with a shock. Third down: Unsuccessful fixed burst pacing. Bottom: Successful ramp pacing termination of ventricular tachycardia

Atrial septal defects

The Amplatzer atrial septal defect occluder has the shape of two saucers connected by a central stent-like cylinder that varies in diameter from 4 mm to 40 mm to allow closure of both small and large atrial septal defects. Very large secundum atrial septal defects with incomplete margins (other than at the aortic end of the defect) may require a surgically placed patch.

An atrial septal defect is sized with catheter balloons of progressively increasing diameter. An occluder of the correct size is then introduced into the left atrium via a long transvenous sheath. The left atrial disk of the occluder is extruded and pulled against the defect. The sheath is then pulled back to deploy the rest of the device (central waist and right atrial disk) and released after its placement is assessed by transoesophageal echocardiography. The defect is closed by the induction of thrombosis on three polyester patches sewn into the device and is covered by neocardia within two months. Aspirin is usually for given for six months and clopidrogrel for 6-12 weeks.

Worldwide, several thousand patients have had their atrial septal defects closed with Amplatzer devices, with high occlusion rates. Complications are unusual and consist of device migration ($<1\%$), transient arrhythmias (1-2%), and, rarely, thrombus formation with cerebral thromboembolism or aortic erosion with tamponade. Transcatheter occlusion is now the treatment of choice for patients with suitable atrial septal defects. Other devices are available, but none has the same applicability or ease of use.

Patent foramen ovale

The Amplatzer atrial septal defect occluder can also be used to treat adults with paradoxical thromboembolism via a patent foramen ovale. The Amplatzer patent foramen ovale occluder has no central stent and is designed to close the flap-valve of the patent foramen ovale. Randomised trials are under way to compare device closure with medical treatment for preventing recurrent thromboembolism.

Patent ductus arteriosus

Although premature babies and small infants with a large patent ductus arteriosus are still treated surgically, most patients with a patent ductus arteriosus are treated by transcatheter coil occlusion. This technique has been highly successful at closing small defects, but when the minimum diameter is >3 mm multiple and larger diameter coils are required, which prolongs the procedure and increases the risk of left pulmonary artery encroachment. The Amplatzer patent ductus arteriosus plug, which has a mushroom shaped Nitinol frame stuffed with polyester, is used for occluding larger defects. The occlusion rates are close to 100%, higher than published results for surgical ligation.

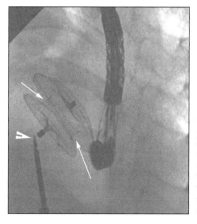

Cineframe showing the three components of the Amplatzer atrial septal defect occluder—a left atrial disk, central stent (arrows), and a right atrial disk. The device has just been unscrewed from the delivery wire, and the male screw on the delivery wire can be seen (arrowhead)

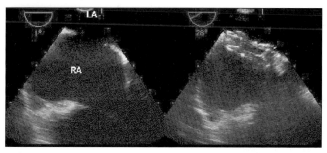

Atrial septal defect occlusion. Transoesophageal echocardiograms of an atrial septal defect before (left) and after (right) occlusion with an Amplatzer atrial septal defect device. The three components of the device are easily seen. (LA=left atrium, RA=right atrium)

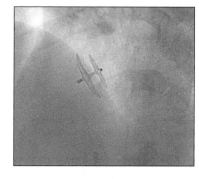

Patent foramen ovale closure. A cine frame of an implanted Amplatzer patent foramen ovale device shows that it differs from the atrial septal defect device in not having a central stent. Its right atrial disk is larger than the left atrial disk and faces in a concave direction towards the atrial septum

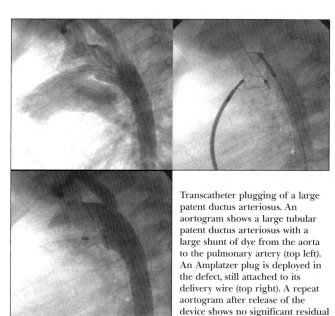

Transcatheter plugging of a large patent ductus arteriosus. An aortogram shows a large tubular patent ductus arteriosus with a large shunt of dye from the aorta to the pulmonary artery (top left). An Amplatzer plug is deployed in the defect, still attached to its delivery wire (top right). A repeat aortogram after release of the device shows no significant residual shunting (left)

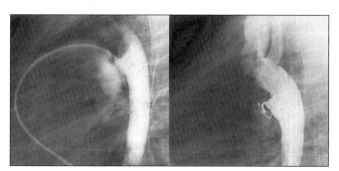

Coil occlusion of a patent ductus arteriosus. An aortogram performed via the transvenous approach shows dye shunting through the small conical patent ductus arteriosus into the pulmonary artery (left). After placement of multiple coils, a repeat aortogram shows no residual shunting (right)

Ventricular septal defects

Occlusion devices are especially useful for multiple congenital muscular ventricular septal defects, which can be difficult to correct surgically. The Amplatzer occluder device has a drum-like shape and is deployed through long sheaths with relatively small diameter.

Such devices have also been used to occlude perimembranous defects, although in this location they can interfere with aortic valve function. A device with eccentric disks, which should avoid interference with adjacent valves, has recently been introduced. The Amplatzer membranous device has two discs connected by a short cylindrical waist. The device is eccentric, with the left ventricular disc having no margin superiorly, where it could come near the aortic valve, and a longer margin inferiorly to hold it on the left ventricular side of the defect. The end screw of the device has a flat portion, which allows it to be aligned with a precurved pusher catheter. This pusher catheter then extrudes the eccentric left ventricular disk from the specially curved sheath with its longer margin orientated inferiorly in the left ventricle. Initial results are promising, particularly for larger infants with haemodynamically important ventricular septal defects.

Transcatheter occlusion has also been used to treat ventricular septal defects in adults who have had a myocardial infarction, and a specific occluder has been introduced. It differs from the infant device in having a 10 mm long central stent to accommodate the thicker adult interventricular septum. Its role in treatment is uncertain, but it offers an alternative for patients who have significant contraindications to surgical closure.

Coil occlusion of unwanted blood vessels

Coil occlusion of unwanted blood vessels (aortopulmonary collateral arteries, coronary artery fistulae, arteriovenous malformations, venous collaterals) is increasingly effective because of improvements in catheter and coil design.

Percutaneous intervention versus surgery

The growth of interventional cardiology has meant that the simpler defects are now dealt with in catheterisation laboratories, and cardiac surgeons are increasingly operating on more complex lesions such as hypoplastic left heart syndrome. More importantly, interventional cardiology can complement the management of these complex patients, resulting in a better outcome for children with congenital heart disease.

Complications such as device embolisation, vessel or chamber perforation, thrombosis, and radiation exposure can be reduced by careful selection of patients and devices, meticulous technique, low dose pulsed fluoroscopy, and, most importantly, operator experience. Further developments in catheter and device design will improve and widen treatment applications.

Competing interests: None declared.

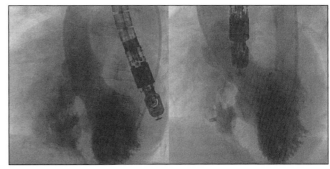

Transcatheter closure of a mid-muscular ventricular septal defect. A left ventriculogram shows substantial shunting of dye through a defect in the mid-muscular ventricular septum (left). After placement of an Amplatzer muscular ventricular septal defect device, a repeat left ventriculogram shows only a small amount of shunting through the device (right), which ceased after three months

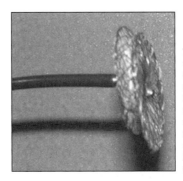

The Amplatzer perimembranous ventricular septal defect device. The two disks are offset from each other to minimise the chance of the left ventricular disk impinging on the aortic valve. The central stent is much narrower than in the muscular ventricular septal defect device as the membranous septum is much thinner than the muscular septum

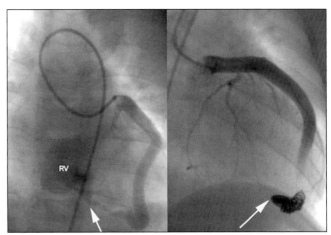

Coil occlusion of a coronary fistula. A selective left coronary arteriogram shows a fistula arising from the left anterior descending coronary artery (arrow, left) draining to the right ventricle (RV). Multiple interlocking detachable coils are placed to completely occlude the fistula (arrow, right)

Further reading

- Kan JS, White RI Jr, Mitchell SE, Gardner TJ. Percutaneous balloon valvuloplasty: a new method for treating congenital pulmonary valve stenosis. *N Engl J Med* 1982;307:540-2
- Waight DJ, Cao Q-L, Hijazi ZM. Interventional cardiac catheterisation in adults with congenital heart disease. In: Grech ED, Ramsdale DR, eds. *Practical interventional cardiology.* 2nd ed. London: Martin Dunitz, 2002:390-406
- Morrison WL, Walsh KP. Transcatheter closure of ventricular septal defect post myocardial infarction. In: Grech ED, Ramsdale DR, eds. *Practical interventional cardiology.* 2nd ed. London: Martin Dunitz, 2002:362-4
- Masura J, Walsh KP, Thanopoulous B, Chan C, Bass J, Goussous Y, et al. Catheter closure of moderate- to large-sized patent ductus arteriosus using the new Amplatzer duct occluder: immediate and short-term results. *J Am Coll Cardiol* 1998;31:878-82
- Walsh KP, Maadi IM. The Amplatzer septal occluder. *Cardiol Young* 2000;10:493-50

Index

Page numbers in **bold** type refer to figures; those in *italics* refer to tables.

Index

The complete ABC series

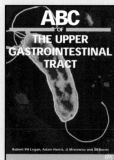

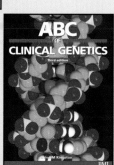

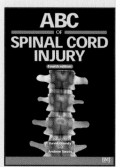

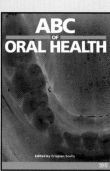

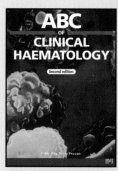

Titles are available from all good medical bookshops or visit:

www.abc.bmjbooks.com